Reverse Parkinson's Disease

by

John Pepper

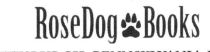

PITTSBURGH, PENNSYLVANIA 15222

First printed under the title 'There Is LIFE After Parkinson's Disease' in The Republic of South Africa in 2003.
Second re-print in The Republic of South Africa in 2009, with the title: 'There is LIFE After Being Diagnosed with Parkinson's Disease'

Website - www.reverseparkinsons.co.za

ISBN: 978-1-4349-8353-4
eISBN: 978-1-4349-4601-0
Printed in the United States of America

First Printing

For more information or to order additional books, please contact:
RoseDog Books
701 Smithfield Street
Pittsburgh, Pennsylvania 15222
U.S.A.
1-800-834-1803
www.rosedogbookstore.com

Contents

For my dear wife, Shirley, whose never ending love and support have encouraged me to believe that I can beat this condition.

Preface

What he will he does, and does so much.
That proof is call'd impossibility.
Shakespeare, Troilus and Cressida, v, 5, 28.

Parkinson's disease is incurable. The disability is chronic and progressive with rising morbidity over a period of time. Medical therapy is the mainstay of conventional treatment. John Pepper has been able to circumvent the standard treatment through his perseverance, original thinking and motivation.

Parkinson's is a syndrome, consisting of a variable combination of tremor, rigidity and bradykinesia (slowness of voluntary movement and an associated reduction in automatic movement, such as swinging of the arms when walking). There is also a characteristic disturbance of gait and posture as well as fixity of facial expression. Although these are the main symptoms there are a multitude of others that John discusses clearly in this book.

John's story is a portrayal of courage, showing the power of focusing on, and being committed to one's beliefs. One can greatly admire his determination and self-motivation, as seen in his conscious efforts to correct and adjust his movements, which in itself is no small achievement. His positive attitude has been further enhanced by the warm and encouraging support of his wife, Shirley and family. This close family relationship has been a positive factor, in helping John cope with his disability has always been, and still is an integral part of his lifestyle, which, combined with the fact that he was fortunate enough to be able to retire from work, have been major lifestyle changes, helping him to cope with stress. At the same time as managing his stress levels, he has been able to control many of the symptoms, by adjusting his diet and his condition has improved considerably. I have always known John to be a very determined person and intent on pushing himself further up the ladder. He has been innovative in his ideas and able to work out subtle and ingenious ways to cope with the difficulties of his condition. All this becomes very obvious as you progress through this book.

I have had the privilege of knowing John and his family for many years and have great admiration for the way in which he has turned his health around and the extent to which he has taken control of his body.

It is my hope that this book will reach many Parkinson's sufferers and serve as a great source of inspiration to them.

Dr Colin Kahanovitz, MB.BCH (Wits)

Acknowledgements

The mere thought of writing a book, especially on something as mystifying as Parkinson's disease, was a very daunting prospect. I offer my thanks and gratitude for everything these people have done to make this book possible:

My dear daughter Diane, who has spent many hours reading and editing numerous drafts of this book, and for all her support, and her family for their contributions.

My family doctor and friend, Dr Colin Kahanovitz, for his loving care and support over many difficult years, and for guiding my thinking, when I was in unknown territory.

To John Telford, the editor of SPRING Times - the Special Parkinson's Research Interest Group's mouthpiece - for all his help and advice, and for all his articles I have been privileged to be allowed to print in this book.

To Bill Bell, the Executive Director of the Northwest Parkinson's Foundation, and for his approval to include many articles from his excellent Northwest Post.

James Byrom, for his permission to include an excerpt from his book, "Fields of Air".

Dr Ian Weinberg for his information on Psychoneuro-immunology (PNI).

Shirley Soll, for encouraging me to extend myself, when I wanted to give up, and for her account of my determination to achieve my goal of improving my personal fitness

Estelle McIlrath, for not accepting that I was unable to draw straight lines, and for her account of my efforts in art.

Adrienne Gruskin, my Parkinson's Support Group leader, who has stood by me, when the going has been quite tough, and for having confidence and belief in me.

My son Sean and his family, for their support and encouragement and for never having been embarrassed, by my un-cool behavior in public.

And finally, I thank my dear wife Shirley, for once again being prepared to spend many hours on her own, while I wrote this book, and who is as committed as I am to changing people's attitudes towards Parkinson's disease.

Introduction

Having Parkinson's disease (Pd) is not the reason for writing this book. Others, more capable than I, have adequately described this condition.

My motivation is far more exciting! **It comes from having been able to reverse most of the more debilitating effects of this movement disorder, and having no further need for Pd medication.** The only medication I now need, in order to treat two of my remaining Pd symptoms, is for insomnia, and until recently, mood swings. However, I do still have many of my Pd symptoms, but I am able to control them in ways that I will explain later. I stopped taking my normal Pd medication in 2003, when I was feeling a great deal better than I had been in 1992, when I was first diagnosed.

As a result of taking a special type of Pd medication and doing regular strenuous exercise, I now live a normal, happy life, no different to most other people.

Why has this happened? This edition, under a new title, contains details of two separate scientifically controlled double blind studies - refer to Appendixes 3 & 4 for more details - the results of which are, in my opinion, responsible for my improved health. The first study confirms that prolonged energetic exercise can slow down, or even reverse, the Pd symptoms. The second study proves that the type of medication I was lucky enough to have been prescribed, can also slow down the progression of Pd, or even reverse it.

I felt that my **good news** should have been welcomed with open arms by the medical profession, but because it hasn't happened before, it has understandably been received with skepticism. It is quite reasonable for the medical profession to be suspicious about my news, although I don't claim to have a cure. Had I have claimed to be cured, then I feel this skepticism would have been justified. As it is, my GP knows my medical history since 1988 and he also knows what sort of person I am. He graciously agreed to write the Preface for the book, and he is as upbeat about my news as I am. I am giving all the information about what happened, after I wrote the first edition, in the chapter titled 'The Aftermath'.

The real mystery is, seeing that there have been **two double blind scientific controlled studies that prove that we can influence the progression of Pd,** of which I assume the medical profession is well aware; then **why is my good news still being met with such skepticism?**

The first piece of my good luck was due to having taken part in prolonged energetic exercise, since the early seventies, after my family and I had moved from the 'diamond' city of Kimberley to the 'gold' city of Springs, close to Johannesburg. My second piece of good luck was having been prescribed with the type of medication referred to in the abovementioned scientific controlled study.

To the best of my knowledge, very few people, possibly including some neurologists, appear to know anything about these two studies. The Parkinson Association South Africa doesn't appear to have been aware of them either. Very few people seem to be aware of them, otherwise I would have expected more interest from neurologists in my Pd history.

These studies were first reported to the public in 2006, long after I set about trying to help myself to beat this condition in 1992, and even when I wrote the first edition of this book in 2002. I had no idea that what I had set about doing could possibly have affected my condition. This was an incredibly lucky happening for me and my family. When I embarked upon my exercise program in the early 70's, it was because of a serious back problem, not because of the Pd symptoms, which had already started to make themselves evident at that time.

I was very fortunate, at the time I was diagnosed, because my neurologist prescribed a single medication (Eldepryl). He told me that the manufacturers claimed it could possibly slow down the progression of Pd. Otherwise, he said, there is no other medication on the market that had been scientifically proven to slow down the progression, and we had to just hope and pray that somebody would come up with a cure in our lifetime. He gave me no other tips about what to do to help ward off the inevitable worsening of my condition. However, he did say that my Pd was still in the early stages. I have subsequently learned that it is not possible to diagnose Pd until approximately 70% of the dopamine producing glial cells in the substantia nigra have been damaged. So, I was already at least 70% down that slippery slope, in 1992.

None of the people with Parkinson's disease (PwP's) I have spoken to, have been prescribed a monotherapy of an MAO-B inhibitor. I am not aware of anybody else, who has been on a prolonged energetic exercise program and has also taken a monotherapy of an MAO-B inhibitor. Both the exercise and the medication have been the subject of controlled scientific studies. Therefore, I strongly feel that my Pd history deserves special investigation and I hope this book will bring this about.

In addition to these two proven factors, the other factors I mention later in the book, such as - **Positive attitude; stress management; brain exercises and a proper eating plan** – have all had, in my opinion, a positive influence on the progression of my Pd. They are generally accepted as being beneficial advice for everybody.

There is another factor, which adds further evidence to the belief that prolonged energetic exercise can slow down or even reverse the progression of Pd. This factor only dawned on me recently, when I was talking to other patients about my Pd experience. My Pd symptoms began back in the early 1960's, but I only started regular energetic exercise in the early seventies. I continued that exercise for the next twenty years, before doctors were able to diagnose the Pd in 1992. It is reasonable to assume that **the exercise must have been slowing down the progression of the PD during that time. Otherwise, the Pd would normally have progressed much quicker.**

After 1992, while taking the medication and doing regular energetic exercise for four years, my health started to improve to the extent that other people noticed an improvement in my condition, even before my family had. Living in close touch with my family, made the slow improvement unnoticeable to them, whereas the people I saw very seldom, noticed immediately. As I say later in the book, I got the distinct impression that these people thought that I had been pulling the wool over their eyes, because everybody knows that **you don't get better, when you have Pd.** I am sure that the medical profession is locked into this mindset!

My daily routine, after having given up my career, consisted of going to the gym for ninety minutes, having a shower and coming home for breakfast. Then, after Shirley went to work, I would relax in a reclining chair, with a book or magazine, listening to classical music on the sound system. In this way I hoped to undo all the damage I had done to my health over the previous thirty years. What happened, more often than not, was that I fell asleep on that chair and, consequently, I was sleeping even worse at night. This, I believe, is a fairly common situation, where PwPs turn day into night. It was not as nice as it may sound. It became rather disturbing for Shirley when, in the middle of the night, I invariably turned on the light, in order to read, until I could drop off to sleep again. My whole idea at the time was to take life easy, and avoid as much stress as possible. I think that this was a very important phase in my overall 'apparent recovery' process, but it was only a temporary situation. Had I gone on much longer, doing very little in the way of regular activity, I think I would have continued to go downhill.

By sharing my experiences with other sufferers, especially those in the early stages of Pd, I hope to help improve their quality of life, by restoring their self confidence and giving them a better understanding of Pd, from a fellow-sufferer's viewpoint.

In order to give you some idea of my background, I was born and educated in England, and immigrated to South Africa in 1952, when I was seventeen years of age.

In 1963, my partner and I established a small printing business in Kimberley, the city of diamonds. This business grew, over thirty odd years, into a much larger business. During this period, my position, as Chairman (President) of that company, slowly developed into a bit of a nightmare.

Being a very ambitious person, I must point out that I never let my ambition take precedence over other aspects of my life. However, that ambition has been an important driving force in my life, and it was responsible for the company's rapid growth. With this growth, came the inevitable business problems, which made my personal life very complicated and difficult.

This situation was self-imposed, and could have been handled very differently to the way I chose, at that time. I am also a compulsive workaholic, and as the company grew, there were many critical periods during which, instead of delegating my workload, I chose to go it alone, until I landed in the situation, where I had no choice but to make changes. However, there was always one part of my responsibility, for which I could not find a suitable person to take over, and that was the writing of programs for my computer, in order to run my business from beginning to end. This reluctance to delegate is a very common failing among entrepreneurs.

After my company listed on the Johannesburg Stock Exchange, in 1987, my abilities and skills as an entrepreneur soon ceased to be appropriate for running a large company. Fortunately, I was aware of my shortcomings, and had already made efforts to find and train a successor, long before the company went public, and before I became aware of having Pd. My symptoms, at that time, were already hampering my ability to function properly as the Chairman of that company.

This inability to professionally manage my company, after it had gone public, had a very important bearing on my illness. It placed me under an enormous amount of **STRESS**.

I am still happily married for the past fifty years (in 2010), to the same wonderful woman. We have two children and six grown-up grandchildren, all of whom have been extremely supportive and understanding over the years.

My gift of improved health is an exciting story and it needs to be told to the whole world, so that others will know what *can* happen, if we don't give up, when things go wrong.

It is not my intention to falsely raise hopes, by leading you to believe that my Pd is cured. I still have most of the symptoms, but they are mostly under control and at a much lower level than they were in 1992.

If you are a fellow PwP, then why not take the time to read this account, and compare your experiences with mine. **No two people's Pd symptoms are the same.** Everybody has a different mix of symptoms. You may have some that I do not mention. Some of the symptoms are those normally associated with Dystonia, which, I believe, is caused in a similar way to Pd, and in the same part of the brain. They are both movement disorders. Other symptoms are also shared with Alzheimer's. All three of these conditions share symptoms with Senility. In other words, it is difficult to know whether some of the symptoms are purely age related or are definitely Pd.

If you are not a PwP, but you do care for someone who is, then my story will possibly shed a new light on the condition. Your encouragement and support is absolutely essential, and without you, the patient could not survive. Occasionally, patients need to be left alone, to muddle through. Sometimes, only a little bit of **prodding** and **encouragement**, are needed, to persuade the patient to embark upon more difficult or sometimes unpleasant activities, which could help make their lives, **and yours**, more bearable.

Part 1

The Reality of Parkinson's

Chapter 1

Why Me?

The shock of being diagnosed with such a daunting disorder was indescribable. The diagnosis came after nearly twenty-five years of health problems, which were treated as individual problems, and not picked up as being part of Pd. My knowledge of Pd, at that time, was limited to my memories of two friends, when they were in the final stages of Pd and exhibiting very disturbing visible symptoms.

My reaction to the diagnosis was naturally, why me? What had I done to bring this about? I am not a big drinker and haven't smoked since I was twenty-seven. Although a little overweight, I am not obese. I have done fairly strenuous exercise for many years. So, **where did I go wrong?**

I do not recall ever hero-worshiping any sports personality, nor was I ever really interested in sport. My disinterest stemmed from having poor to average muscle coordination and a resultant inferior sporting ability. My eyesight has been very poor, since childhood. Early on in life I made the erroneous assumption that sporting ability is something you either have at birth, or you don't. I knew I didn't have it, and felt I was forever doomed to mediocrity in the sporting world. So, in my ignorance, I assumed that sporting heroes inherited their abilities, and therefore did not warrant the excessive adulation poured upon them.

I did not realize when I was young, that playing sport is essential for the development of the body, and the mind. It isn't winning games that is important, it is learning to enjoy the game and the interaction with other people.

The same applied to academia. Why try to compete with people, who have superior brains? Our brains all need to develop, the same as our bodies, so listening to these people, thinking about what they say, and taking in what we understand, must help us to develop. The best way to get the benefit of other people's knowledge and experience is to read

14

books. I never read a book from cover to cover, as a young person, other than at school, until I was married, in 1960. I had a reading problem, when I was young, and had to concentrate so hard on the reading that I did not take in the content of *what* I was reading. Therefore, I didn't enjoy it.

As I grew older, I began to realize that we could be very gifted at birth and yet achieve nothing in our lives. So, contrary to my immature beliefs, I later realized that there *is* a lot to admire, if people are able and prepared to nurture the gifts nature has bestowed upon them, and get to the top in their chosen fields of endeavor. We are all given certain abilities, and disabilities, at birth, and it is what we choose to do with those abilities, and how we try to overcome those disabilities, which determines what we make of our lives.

Why I mention this is; after being diagnosed, I *did* become very influenced by the extraordinary achievements of two very special people. At that time, I desperately needed to take strength from others, who had managed to do the seemingly impossible.

The first of these icons was Helen Keller, who, although having been born deaf, dumb and blind, managed to overcome those daunting impediments, to become a world-renowned pioneer in specialized communication skills. Her story is an example to everybody.

The second icon was Douglas Bader, who lost both his legs in a plane crash, while showing off, soon after having learned how to fly. He desperately wanted to become a pilot again, but knew that unless he could walk, unaided, he would never be accepted as a pilot. So, he taught himself to walk properly, on **two artificial legs,** without the aid of crutches or walking sticks. He also managed to persuade his senior officers to let him fly a fighter plane again, and later became a renowned war hero.

This all took a great deal of courage and determination, on both their parts, and they have been an inspiration to me in my adult life. I have learned from them that:

There is no limit to what our minds and bodies are capable of achieving, if we want something badly enough. *They* had no unusual inherited skills or aptitude, so **what made them special?**

Douglas Bader was not born any different to most of us. He just had such tremendous **determination and courage.**

15

Being deaf dumb and blind is not the best start to have in life, and if anybody could be excused for non-achievement, Helen Keller could. What she needed, and later found, from somebody else, was a great deal of **self-belief**!

Over the years, I have discovered that I have a few artistic abilities, including acting, singing, painting and sculpting. These abilities did not come to the fore all at once, and even when they did, I did absolutely nothing to develop any of them; I was always too busy. When I found that I was capable of acting, I *was very tempted* to take it up as a career, but that had too many drawbacks attached to it. My family was, and still is, a very important part of my life, and being away from home, attending endless rehearsals and performances, became a serious problem in our marriage.

Instead of acting, I chose to go into business, in partnership with a good friend, and then later on, with another like-minded entrepreneur. This gave my family the opportunity to - live in a comfortable home; actively take part in rewarding community service; send our two children to good schools and universities; see them both become very well-balanced citizens, successful in their chosen careers; help them raise their own families; and enjoy life to the full.

Maybe, one man does not deserve to have so much happiness and success. I certainly did not deserve to have so many talents, and I am often ashamed that I did not do more to develop most of them. Maybe, I just needed to have a taste of hardship and real problems, as other people have, to make me appreciate all the privileges I have in life.

The arrival of Parkinson's disease in my life has certainly taught me a few bitter lessons. I have had to accept that I can no longer present to the world, the same confident person I once was. I have had to accept that my memory isn't what it used to be and my word vocabulary doesn't function properly, when I address meetings, or even when I talk to friends.

Shirley and I have kept our relationships alive, over the years, with the friends we have made, during our married life. We have continued to meet with this wide circle of friends, since we set out on our journey together. These friends all know what sort of person I am. They don't react badly, when they see me spill wine, or fall over. I am still the same person I always have been, before I contracted this terrible affliction, and I don't have to prove anything to them. I have been open and up-front with them all about my Pd. I didn't pretend that there was nothing wrong, and they accepted my need to sleep at odd times, and my apparent disinterest in the general conversation.

When I was diagnosed in 1992, I was convinced that the doctor must have made a mistake. I am not alone in having had this conviction. I think it was part of the initial process of **denial and mourning**. I could not accept that I had to, "Get used to the fact of having Pd, and get on with my life". I had not yet given in to the inevitability of Pd.

I did get on with my life, but not in the way the neurologist had in mind. After a two-year period of introspection, I decided to **take charge of my life,** once more...

I slowly set about examining my lifestyle. I soon began making very necessary changes in **the way I thought**, and in my **attitude towards life**. I found at that stage that **I had allowed myself to become a victim**, when I had always thought of myself as a winner. What had changed, and when? I had become so engrossed in the problems related to my work, that I had not taken any notice of my declining health. I had managed to **push aside** the discomforts and peculiar experiences I was increasingly encountering.

I decided, after those first two years, to start doing anything I could to possibly stave off the inevitable progression of Pd. As a movement disorder, I assumed that the more I moved, the slower the Pd would be able to take over my life. On the one hand, I was already going to the gym for one and a half hours, six days of the week, and did not have the energy, or will, to do any more. On the other hand, I was sitting around, doing nothing active, for the rest of those two years.

I realized that I had slowly removed myself from society. I did not mix with anybody at the gym, and I had ceased seeing anybody during this two-year period, other than close family. This was not normal. People do not normally withdraw from life, while still reasonably young!

Having realized that only *I* could bring about a change in my life, I had to ask myself;

What did I have to do to change this situation?

The answer turned out to be quite simple! I had to change my **attitude**.

Why had I become a victim? Was it the diagnosis? No! My attitude, at the time of the diagnosis, was no better than it had been, many years earlier. It had gradually changed during the mid-seventies, at about the time I was diagnosed with depression. I realize now that I had already ceased being positive, long before I was diagnosed with Pd. That was a very crucial stage of my life. I had to recognize the fact that I had allowed matters in the workplace to get out of hand, I wasn't sleeping, and I had ceased doing anything constructive in my private life. My life had become full of incredible problems, and those problems needed resolution.

In addition to my responsibilities as Chairman of a fast growing company, I was very involved, for thirteen years, with Round Table, which is a worldwide organization of young men, united in the ideals of service to the community. At the age of Forty, I was compelled to leave that organization, which has an age-limit of 40. I soon joined Rotary International, and spent the next fourteen years with them, and served as President and District Governor's Representative. At around the time of being President of the Rotary club, I was also elected as President of my local Master Printers Association, for two years. You can imagine how much extra pressure these commitments put upon my shoulders. All of these activities added even more work to my already overworked schedule. With the benefit of hindsight, I was foolish to have gotten involved with any of these organizations, but we all need some outside activities, but through them, I grew very much as a person.

Having already given up working, three months after diagnosis, I found that I had not got rid of all the baggage I was carrying around with me. I was still worrying about what I should, and could, have done to extricate myself from the computer programming; not realizing that it was all in the past, and of no consequence. I had to learn to accept that:

What was, was, and **What is, is**!

Only at that point in my life, did I slowly set about becoming more positive. When I took stock of myself, I realized that I could still walk, albeit, rather awkwardly. I could still travel. Shirley and I were still good friends, as well as lovers. We could still enjoy our life together; but only if I was prepared to give up all those negative thoughts and **allow myself** to enjoy life again. Shirley had plenty of misgivings about our future, but she did not share them with me. Outwardly, she stayed very positive and supportive.

Why my condition had improved to such an extent in 2002, at the time of writing the first edition of this book, I was not able to say with absolute certainty? But **that situation has now changed**. Although, what I have to tell you is not only perfectly true, it is also mainly common sense. This is why I am anxious to tell you my story, to see whether others can benefit from that experience.

My huge improvement has become a bit of an enigma to me. Because I look so well, some neurologists have taken one look at me and said, 'You obviously don't have Pd' and 'you should not go around telling other people that you do have Pd.

I suppose this viewpoint is understandable. **Getting better** is unheard of in Pd patients. They always **get worse.** This dogmatic attitude is such a pity because, if we close our minds to the **probability that I do indeed have Pd**, and what I have been doing *appears to have* **helped my brain to repair itself**; then we will lose the opportunity to learn something new and exciting.

If people don't *believe* that I have Pd, because doctors are telling them that I don't, then:

Everything I have learned and everything that has happened to me will all be lost forever.

At the time of writing this third edition, the benefits of meaningful exercise **have already been backed up by research,** which came to the fore in 2006, details of which are quoted in Appendixes 3 and 4.

Further information may be found at the following websites: SPRING Seminar on the Benefits of Exercise as a Pd Therapy: http://tinyurl.com/pd-exercise
Exercise for Pd – The evidence under scrutiny:
http://spring.parkinsons.org.uk/springdocs/NieuwboerPage.html
Exercise and Pd – evidence for efficacy from cellular and animal studies:
http://spring.parkinsons.org.uk/springdocs/ZigmondPage.html

To finish off, I have to return to the question posed in the title of this chapter: Why Me?

Well! Why not?

Chapter 2

The GOOD News

My good news is;

With determination and self-belief, I am sure that many of us can turn the tables on Pd.

When I became a PwP, I did not immediately set out to beat the condition, like some intrepid pioneer. I knew nothing about the subject, and from what I had heard, on that nightmare day of diagnosis, I was distinctly under the impression that there *was nothing I could* do about it, even if I wanted to. I have **found nothing**, **about which, the medical profession didn't already know,** but I have dealt with the Pd in a very different way to most others. My story *should be* very interesting, especially to newly diagnosed patients.

My experiences should shed some new light on the subject of movement disorders, and should give my fellow sufferers some much-needed **hope for the future.**

Unfortunately, I have the feeling that, due to the nature of the disease, the mind-set of many longer-term PwPs is so negative, that they may find it very difficult to believe that they could *possibly* bring about an improvement in their condition. However, I still believe in miracles, and that **nothing is impossible**. I only have **to convince you** of this possibility. Having just learned to swim, did you ever wonder why you thought you couldn't do it in the first place? Nothing had changed! You had only **overcome the fear of drowning.**

Many of us do not have enough time to wait for new treatments, and especially not a cure. In the meantime, our condition slowly but surely continues to deteriorate, and we become more rigid, and dependent upon others to help us get through each day. Since I first became aware of Pd, In 1960, there has not been that one announcement, for which we all so fervently pray, that a cure has been found for Pd.

My news relates to my own experience, since I was diagnosed, and because I am not unique, I believe that what has happened to me, *can* happen to others. On the face of it, my assessment, when I wrote the first edition, was that it would not cost the patient any money to make this lifestyle change, which would have been very nice for the patients. However, with the benefit of several years, talking to patients, since that first book was published, I have to accept that the average person is not going to do regular exercise, unless it is an organized activity. Very few PwP's have the drive to go out alone, at a regular time every other day, in order to participate in regular exercise. This needs to be an organized activity, with a professional overseeing that nobody gets injured and that everybody does the correct amount of exercise, at a correct level. The obvious choice for this supervision would be a biokineticist. Also, the provision of a range of suitable brain exercises needs some entrepreneurial skills. It is not going to cost a fortune, and should be a cheaper and healthier alternative to total reliance on medication, of which it is hoped you will need less, the more you exercise.

I have not invented a new gadget, which you can run out and buy. I have not come across a previously unknown chemical, which I could put into pill form, to pop into your mouth, three times a day. As I have already said, what I have discovered **has been known to medical science for a long time**, but that knowledge does not appear to have filtered down to the people dealing with Parkinson's disease.

What I am going to recommend to you, only requires your time, a certain amount of energy, some possible discomfort and a lot of **self-motivation and commitment.**

I suspect that the medical profession is dubious about the benefits of doing what I have done. I get the distinct impression that they feel that it is too simple, too glib. But, the results speak for themselves. Sometimes, simple solutions are the best. What I am advocating may appear to be simple, but it requires a lot of commitment and determination to pull it off. If my experience proves to work for everybody, as it already appears to have done for some, then these theories *should* have a very beneficial effect upon the way the medical profession treats Pd patients in the future. Biokineticists will have the opportunity to approach the treatment of Pd patients in very different ways to those of the past.

In 1992, I had to face up to the reality of ***Parkinson's disease***. At that stage, I had already **lost my self-confidence**. I was experiencing difficulty performing many of my daily tasks, which I had taken for-granted, all my life. The indignity, of having to ask Shirley, or my children, to help me perform simple mundane tasks, like fastening my buttons, tying my shoelaces or putting on my socks, was something with which I could not come to terms. I seemed to have no proper control over my fingers at all, with the result that they were incapable of performing any fine motor functions, when I needed them most. My speech sometimes made me sound as if I had imbibed a little too much and my walk was that of a much older man.

My list of medical problems, in those days, was not confined to Pd, in fact, that was probably the least of my worries, at the time, although it obviously had the makings of a far worse situation later on.

I have suffered for many years with severe back problems, which seemed to come and go without any warning. I finally had a disc removed from my lower spine (Laminectomy), in 1977, and because I carried on with my life, as if there were nothing wrong, I had to expect a few episodes of lumbar pains. I also contracted Meniere's Syndrome in the early seventies, which has left me with considerably reduced hearing in my left ear, and perpetual tinnitus, since 1985. This alone was enough to ruin even the most beautiful day. The giddiness fits, which are often accompanied by vomiting and headaches, are very intermittent, but very debilitating, when they happen.

In addition to these, not insignificant problems, I had what was then thought to have been osteoarthritis, in my shoulders and knees; an ectopic heart condition; high blood pressure; high cholesterol; asthma; lactose intolerance and other allergy problems. So, you have a picture of a seemingly not-too-healthy person. Although, I have never thought of myself as a sickly person, and don't intend to start now.

What would you expect, from someone who regularly worked more than sixteen hours a day and slept for an average of less than four hours a night, since 1974?

My medical bills were enormous. These alone should have been enough incentive for me to stop and take a hard look at what I was doing to myself but, like many others, I was too busy to see what was really happening to me.

The truth is; *I was too BUSY to be sick.* I have always regarded myself as a healthy person, although the above list of problems paints a very different picture. In contrast to my situation, I have met people who had nothing apparently wrong with them, but who regarded themselves as far from healthy. It is **all in the mind,** really! Busy people don't have time to give in to the odd aches and pains, and when they do, they get over it as quickly as possible. Most mothers know what I am talking about.

Eventually, it was the shock of being told that I had an incurable degenerative neurological disease that would gradually make me totally immobile, which made me sit up and listen to what my body had been trying to tell me. It was the realization that I was already on that slippery slope, which made me sit up and take notice, before it was too late.

I have often been reminded of those old clichés, "When you take your hand out of a bucket of water, **you don't leave a hole behind**" and, "**Nobody is indispensable!**" Nevertheless, I was obsessed with the need to complete my life's tasks.

After receiving that fateful diagnosis and deciding to give up my job; it took me three months to give up everything that needed my attention, on a daily basis, and to hand over my main responsibility of running the printing business to my successor. I then closed down the separate computer software company, which was giving me most of my headaches.

Why did I wait so long?

Looking back now, I am amazed that I did not pack it in sooner. My family was suffering, even more than I was. In fact, I was lucky to still have a family. I was even luckier to have received their full support, when they were faced with the daunting prospect of having to care for me for the rest of my life. They did not flinch from the idea that I was likely to need washing, dressing and feeding, on a regular basis. Even the prospect, of having to regularly clean up the mess, when I became incontinent, did not deter them.

What a lucky man I am. While I was working those long hours it wasn't me who was suffering, it was my family. After all those years of neglect, they were still prepared to rally around me, in my hour of need.

There were obviously compensations for the lack of my presence in their lives, during those years, but money and possessions cannot compensate for lack of companionship and non-attendance at important family functions.

Fortunately for me, I never worked over weekends, and we have always remained a close-knit family. Those cherished weekends together were our saving grace.

That is not all my good news.

Other than not needing to take any more Pd medication, walking, without any sign of a bad gait, is now a reality, unless I am **tired**, or **not concentrating**. Making a fool of myself, at mealtimes, by regularly spilling my food or wine, is now only a painful memory, although it still happens on odd occasions. Yes, contrary to all advice about the harmful effects of alcohol, I do occasionally drink wine with the odd meal. When I say "occasionally", I mean about once a week. I also occasionally drink a whisky in the evening, before dinner, but seldom when I know that I am going to have wine with the meal. This is a little more than once a week.

Shirley no longer has to fasten or unfasten my shirt buttons or help me with the odd dressing and undressing problems, like pulling on my socks. Sleeping at night is still a problem, although it tends to be a lot better, now that I take Trepiline. Now, unless I am tired or stressed; I seldom fall asleep during the daytime; my voice still disappears, for no apparent reason; I no longer slur my words or struggle to form sentences, which is probably more to do with concentrating now, on what I want to say. I still choke on food and liquids, which seem to run down my throat, while I am still breathing. I also occasionally have difficulty initiating a swallow. I still find it difficult to swallow certain food items, such as potatoes, well-done meat, dry sandwiches and pumpkin. I cannot remember the last time that I dribbled on my pillow. I can live with the odd occasion, when I get the sudden urge to urinate, or when I think I want to urinate, but can't.

Why? What has changed?

At the time of writing the first edition of this book, I did not know, with any certainty whatsoever, what had brought about these improvements in my **overall condition**. However, I was fully aware of every single experiment I had carried out, since 1992, some of which *had* helped me to improve my quality of life. *Why* had these actions brought about this change in my overall condition? **I am now in the position to be able to say for certain,** although, at the time I embarked upon my attempt to beat Pd, I did not know. I developed my own theories, as I went along, of what I thought needed to be done, some of which were possibly only *pie-in-the-sky* but, most of these theories have turned out to be good.

What were these theories?

Other than exercise, positive thinking and the management of stress; one of my theories was based on a seminar I attended in 1998, led by Doctor Ian Weinberg, a well-known local neurosurgeon. He believes that many diseases, like cancer, are often **triggered** by a traumatic event in the patient's life. He believes it is at this point that some people cease being able to cope with life's problems, and they unknowingly go into decline. The first body function to be affected by this decline is the **immune system**, which ceases to function properly, thereby opening the floodgates to progressively more serious infections and diseases, until the body eventually succumbs.

This appears to be the body's way of dealing with unresolved trauma. The most common traumatic events in our lives are:

i)   The death of a loved one
ii)   Divorce
iii) Retrenchment
iv) Retirement
v)   A Serious accident
vi)   Bankruptcy

There is no doubt that my situation, since I started my own business, had become very traumatic indeed, although the trauma itself could not, and did not, cause my Pd. If Dr Weinberg is correct in his beliefs, and I had in fact been traumatized by not being able to cope with my job, then I felt that it was possible that **my body was reacting to that trauma by reducing the effectiveness of my immune system.**

Dr Weinberg also believes that people first have to come to terms with their trauma, before they can treat any resultant illness. Only when they have succeeded in coming to terms with the trauma, can their bodies *start* once more to cope. The immune system can then regenerate itself. The body can then start to heal itself, as it has been doing throughout our lives. We all carry cancer cells in our bodies, so why don't we all get cancer? The answer is; our immune systems constantly fight disease, without our even being aware.

What Dr. Weinberg is saying makes sense, although he has, as yet, no definite proof. Dr Lori Manson, a senior clinical consultant at my, then, Medical Aid Society, pointed out that Dr Weinberg's theory is based on speculation and that no empirical, evidence-based studies have been done to prove the link between a traumatic experience and the onset of serious illness. Dr Weinberg was very emphatic that trauma cannot cause Pd, because the deterioration in the brain cannot be caused by a failing immune system. However, I was not looking for the cause of my problems, when I went to his seminar. I was looking for a way to deal with my Pd situation.

I have definitely found that stress does influence the progression of Pd, and when I have been able to remove whatever has stressed me, from time to time, my condition had improved.

Another of my theories was that giving up my work, and the consequent reduction of pressure on my mind and body, had an immediate beneficial effect on my health. It is reasonable to assume that the stress my work created, was contributing to my overall health problems, but that does not mean it was necessarily traumatic, but it was stressful. I definitely feel my body was unable to handle that stress any longer.

With the benefit of hindsight, it is quite probable I *could* have achieved the same results much sooner, by removing the causes of my stress, long before the Pd.

Not everyone is fortunate enough to be able to give up work, and I would not recommend this radical step, even be considered, unless it is obvious there is no other alternative. If I were faced with the choice between either continuing to work and increase my wealth, while my health slowly deteriorated, or, giving up that work and income, thereby allowing my body a chance to recuperate, I know which decision I would still make, but it is easy to be wise in hindsight.

If you think about this choice for a moment, you will realize, as I did, that my state of health was not good and, unless I made *changes to my lifestyle,* it would be reasonable to expect my health to continue deteriorating.

From 1974, when I purchased my first computer, up until the time I retired, I was used to getting up as early as three o'clock on most mornings, and working on my computer. I seemed to be unable to sleep after that time, even in the absence of any really pressing issues.

During that period 1974 to 1987, I had been accustomed to working at home at night, writing computer programs, which were urgently needed to run my business. During the day I commuted over fifty kilometers each way to my factory, after having loaded my rather cumbersome computer, together with the bulky disc drive and printer into my car, at one end, and having unloaded them again at the other end. These programs had to be constantly upgraded over the years, in order to keep pace with computer developments, which made the computers faster and more flexible. My business came to depend one hundred percent upon these programs and, consequently, if they had not worked properly, then my business would have ground to a halt. You all know what happens when the computers are out of action at your bank - everything comes to a standstill! Nothing can happen, until they manage to get the monsters up and running again. The same applied to my business.

The pressures on me were sometimes unbearable, especially when I had made changes, which did not work properly. Unfortunately for me, I am the type of person who does not know when he is beaten. I was always so close to reaching the solution to my problems, that I could never have dreamed throwing in the towel. This sounds a little melodramatic, but it is true.

Can you imagine not being able to sleep for more than four hours, on most nights, for over twenty years? My family was just waiting, one day, for me to keel over, due to exhaustion, but somehow that never happened. There are many people in all sorts of occupations, including doctors and mothers, who know very well what it is like to live without sleep, and still be expected to do their jobs properly the next day. So I was not alone. In fact, I was in very good company.

You may well ask, "Why did you not get someone else to write the programs?" This is difficult to answer, objectively. In those days, the combination of the intimate knowledge of printing, and the printing industry, together with the specialized knowledge of running a printing business and the very rare ability, in those days, to write computer programs, was not to be found anywhere. I had all that knowledge and ability, and once I had embarked on this project, there was no turning back. On the bright side, my company was very successful, as was witnessed by its listing on the Johannesburg stock exchange in 1987.

I only mention this in order to give you some idea as to what pressure I had allowed myself to be put under. There was no turning back, other than at enormous expense, and the risk of delays, which could conceivably have crippled my business. It was easier to find a manager for the business than it was to find a programmer, who had the necessary intricate knowledge of the printing industry. In fact, long before I retired, I had already worked myself out of my job.

However bad the work situation had become, as stated earlier, I made a point of never working at weekends, because this was my family time. After having worked over eighty hours during the week, I felt that I did not need to work over the weekends as well. By the time our children had left home and the business had gone public, I found it judicious to make an exception to this rule. Whenever Shirley and I were at home on a Sunday, and I could not sleep, I used to creep out of bed, in the middle of the night, and go into my study. There I would put in six or seven hours work, before taking Shirley a wake-up-cup of coffee. She did not mind me working, while she was enjoying her sleep, as in most instances, she was not even aware of my having been up. This was not stressful to me. In fact, it was a pleasure, because I did my best work early in the morning, and it was better than tossing and turning in bed, while my mind mulled over all the problems, which needed attention, or the solutions to the program problems. I found that I was able to think of solutions to program problems, while still in the process of waking up, and then, when I was ready to get up, I went to my computer and wrote good code.

Here is another theory: If the immune system is controlled by the brain, and the brain can instruct the immune system to 'Shut down', when the body cannot cope with a traumatic situation, then it is possible that the brain can also prematurely initiate some of the ageing processes as well, when it can no longer cope with stress. To the best of my knowledge, some of the symptoms of Pd are possibly linked in some way to that aging process. This is pure conjecture on my part.

The good news is, regardless of whether or not my theories had any merit, my health has improved so much over an eighteen-year period (up to 2010) that:

I no longer *appear* to have Pd.

Having written many letters in our Parkinson's newsletter, without receiving one single reply; could it be that:

- The minds of my fellow PwPs are closed to any positive news about Pd.
- We are conditioned to believe that nothing can be done about Pd?
- We are so negative, in our outlook, that we are not even prepared to contemplate a possible way of halting or reversing this process.

If I were in another person's shoes, I would probably be very skeptical about a claim, whereby a change of lifestyle can bring about a radical improvement in my Pd symptoms, and my overall well being, especially if that claim comes from a non-medical person. **If that claim had been made by my doctor, or a scientist, I would have probably given it more credence**.

You may well ask, 'How is it possible for an old man of seventy-five (in mid 2010), to come up with a way of overcoming some of the more visible effects of Pd, to such an extent that he no longer appears to have Pd?'

The only answer to this hypothetical question is that, as a PwP, it is easier to know what works and what doesn't. We are not all in the position to experiment with medicines, and the only other way we can help ourselves is to play around with our diets, physical activities and mental attitudes. Other than MAO-B inhibitors, there are, to the best of my knowledge, no other medications on the market, that the manufacturers have positively claimed can slow down or reverse Pd. Most Pd medications temporarily hide some of the symptoms, but do not affect the progression of the Pd.

If the improvement in my health is purely the result of the change in my daily lifestyle, then there is not a great deal of opportunity for anyone, other than certain therapists, to develop this knowledge into a lucrative business. However, I have no doubt whatsoever that, **unless the medical profession finds a way to encourage PwPs to adopt the necessary lifestyle changes, which I will elaborate upon later, then, very few PwPs will ever benefit from this news at all.** Taking medicine is a lot easier than changing lifestyles and, because old habits tend to die hard, making such a change, is not going to be easy. In order to change any habit, such as smoking, or giving up drugs, people have first got to make up their minds that they **really *want* to make that change.**

This is the secret! It sounds easy, doesn't it?

Ask any smoker or drug addict, "How easy it is to give up their habit?" The answer is that it obviously is not. So, no, it is not going to be easy to do what I am going to suggest.

You may be wondering why the negativity. Well, I am a realist, and I have no illusions whatsoever about the difficulties involved in changing the way people think.

However, I know that some other PwPs have already been **motivated** enough to make the necessary lifestyle changes, in order to improve their quality of life. I tend to believe that it has proved to be far more difficult for PwPs, whose condition has deteriorated to the stage, where they have limited movement. The side effects of medication are fairly pronounced, and these could also be making the necessary changes to PwP's lifestyle very difficult. I hope that I am wrong in this assessment.

If other PwPs *are* able to duplicate my efforts, with the same result, *then* it will be clear to everybody that we are onto something very substantial indeed. With this in mind, I have tried to persuade the Special Parkinson's Research Interest Group (SPRING) to push for a Controlled Study on the two main tenets of my theory, that the combination of an MAO-B inhibitor and a three-times a week 'Energetic Walking Program' can have a very beneficial effect on Pd. They have pointed out that they are not in the position to motivate controlled studies, but they can advise me on the way to go about it. So far, I have not been able to come up with a practical way in which this could be done. So, I have reluctantly given up hope of successfully motivation such a study. This is not surprising, as I am not a scientist.

I have even found it quite difficult to persuade other PwP's to do exactly what I have done, mainly because I am in no position to instruct doctors to prescribe an MAO-B inhibitor, instead of other medications. But, there are other possible reasons why I have not been all that successful in persuading others to follow my lead:

1. Many, if not all PwPs, suffer from depression. This is a common symptom of Pd, and I don't know if any of us is ever really free of it. This does not mean that it is not *possible* to motivate people with depression. I am saying that I have not so far been very successful in doing so. When someone cannot see light at the end of the tunnel, it

could mean that he or she is looking in the wrong direction. If our Pd was triggered by undue stress, which was directly related to lifestyle, then maybe we should be **retracing our steps?**

2. It is possible that the Pd has progressed beyond the point, where an energetic recovery program would be pointless.

3. Perhaps some **PwPs don't really *want*** to get better. Here I have to be brutally honest. After diagnosis, I fell into the trap of **feeling very sorry for myself.** I clearly remember that during my first year, after diagnosis, I began to enjoy the luxury of being waited upon, for my every need, and being spoilt rotten. I enjoyed not having to make an excuse to lie down and sleep, or sit and read a book and listen to music. I enjoyed the sympathy that was being lavished upon me, by my family and friends. I began to cherish the fact that I no longer had to run around like a madman. There comes a time in our lives, when we long to just let go, which might be part of the body's 'Shutting down' process. I know that we would all *like* to feel better, but that is entirely different to *wanting* **to make the effort to make it happen**.

One of the many lessons I have learned in life, was handed down to me, in 1957, by a casual girlfriend who, upon hearing me say that I would love to be able to play the piano, asked me why I didn't take piano lessons. *OOPS!* She also said that I was only paying lip service to my desires and that was not going to turn my wishes into reality; or words to that effect.

When I started out on my quest to change my attitude, I was doing it to improve *my quality of life,* which, due to my rigidity and clumsiness, was fast becoming untenable. There was no thought of trying to prolong my life. I had been abusing my body for nearly forty years, and I was determined to try to make amends for my stupidity, albeit, after the horse had left the proverbial stable. I had no idea that it was going to improve my overall condition.

Unfortunately, I think that if I offered a miracle pill to achieve the same results, I would find plenty of takers and would have to beat them off with a stick. When movement is so difficult, **the last thing we need is someone telling us to do a lot of exercise**, regardless of what the goal is.

My awareness of Pd is first hand. I am well aware of the paralyzing fear it strikes into the minds of sufferers, when they first hear they have Pd. I am also well aware of what it does to the lives of those wonderful caregivers, who are possibly more affected by the Pd than we are.

Consequently, I am determined to share the knowledge I have gained, with other sufferers. Why am I **not claiming to be cured**, if no one would ever know that I have Pd? Well, I still have many symptoms, which do not improve and some, which lurk in the background, waiting for me to relax my guard. The symptoms are not very debilitating, but I would prefer not to have any at all. I am the last person to make the claim of a cure, even though I doubt that any neurologist would detect any signs of Pd, if I did not volunteer any information. (Refer to Part 4)

Although I still have quite a few Pd symptoms, none of which, other than choking, cause me any real problems in my daily life; my quality of life is as good as any other person of my age. For my part, all it has taken is:

- The *right medication*
- *A lot of time*
- *A great deal of effort*
- A *positive attitude*
- *Management of harmful stress*
- *The good sense to have stopped working*

Read on to find out *HOW this has happened* to me, and how *you* can possibly improve *your own* quality of life, and that of those around you.

Only *YOU* can help to improve your own quality of life. Medication can help to temporarily facilitate your movements and bodily functions, but *YOU* have to do all the other things, in order to help your body to function properly, and *YOU* have to become positive about yourself, and your future.

Part 2

The Process of Achieving My Improved Condition

Foreword

Although there have already been many controlled studies on exercise, it appears that the medical profession is not convinced by the studies already done. Why, I do not know. They appear to want more studies, to prove conclusively that the brain does, in fact, repair itself, when we do energetic exercise. We might also need to prove the benefits of the other claims made on the previous page. I don't think this is necessary, bearing in mind all that has been written about them in the past..

I would like to recommend a book to you entitled, "The Brain that Changes Itself", written by Dr Norman Doidge[1], who is a Canadian psychiatrist, researcher and expert on neuroplasticity.

"This book is about the revolutionary discovery that the human brain can change itself, as told through the stories of the scientists, doctors, and patients, who have together brought about these astonishing transformations. Without operations or medications, they have made use of the brain's hitherto unknown ability to change. Some were patients, like me, who had what were thought to be incurable brain problems; others were people without specific problems who simply wanted to improve the functioning of their brains or preserve them as they aged.

For four hundred years, this venture would have been inconceivable because mainstream medicine and science believed that brain anatomy was fixed. The common wisdom was that after childhood, the brain changed only when it began the long process of decline; that when brain cells failed to develop properly, or were injured, or died, they could not be

---

[1] *Published by Viking, New York, (2007), Preface page.*

replaced. Nor could the brain ever alter its structure and find a new way to function, if part of it was damaged. The theory of the unchanging brain decreed that people who were born with brain or mental limitations, or who sustained brain damage, would be limited or damaged for life. Scientists, who wondered if the healthy brain might be improved or preserved through activity or mental exercise, were told not to waste their time."

These are the words of Dr Doidge himself.

Although I believe this has happened to my brain, I cannot presume to claim that belief to be true.

An accident, which happened in 1961, has had a profound effect on my Parkinson's story. In 1960, I was asked to take the lead part in a production of an old musical titled 'The Arcadians'. In this part, I had to sing and dance, as well as act. I had never danced on stage before, or since. At one stage in the first act, I had to lift the leading lady into the air. Being newly married, and having my wife present, in the chorus, I was very shy, and was reluctant to hold this attractive young lady too close to my body, as I lifted her up in the air. In fact, I held her at arm's length, which is not good for the back, and as I lifted her, we all heard a loud crack, and I dropped her like a stone. What had happened was the pressure exerted on the lower spine, had ruptured a disc.

This has caused me a great deal of pain and suffering over the years. What has this got to do with Pd? Well! In the years that followed this accident I went to several doctors about my back and leg pains, but nobody was able to rectify the problem. In 1968, I was advised by one neurosurgeon to visit a chiropractor, which I did immediately. He told me that the only thing that would help my problem was to strengthen the muscles in my back, to protect the spine. I started gym in 1969 and regular jogging in 1970. Sixteen years after injuring my back, in 1977, my neurosurgeon felt that back surgery had improved to the point where the chances of a successful removal of the disc were very good, and the risks were minimal.

After I had the operation in 1977, I came out of hospital on the third day, and sang on stage that evening and the next, at my daughter's annual dancing display. Since then I have continued to run or walk regularly, and also continued the gym until 1994. All this exercise was done to keep my back strong, but it also appears to have helped keep my Pd at bay. My first symptoms of Pd occurred in the early to mid 60's, and others followed over the years, leading up to the diagnosis in 1992.

That injury on stage in 1961 has, in my humble opinion, been mainly responsible for my good health today, because it had necessitated my doing regular energetic exercise ever since. It is therefore my opinion that this exercise regimen enabled my brain to slow down the progression of the Pd until 1992, when it was finally diagnosed.

The lifestyle changes I made after the initial 'mourning period', between 1992 and 1994, are listed in Appendix 1. I hope that this will encourage other PwPs to change their lifestyles, and do what I have done, and hopefully derive the same benefits. Remember, I cannot influence your doctor's prescription for your medication. Only you can do that!

There was no preconceived plan of action on my part, against which I could have measured my progress. In fact, when I decided to write this book, I had to think very hard about everything that had changed in my life, since diagnosis, and then assess which of these changes have, in my opinion, been beneficial.

In order to present a coherent story, I have broken it down into six separate aspects of my life, which I felt had a bearing on my deteriorating health at the time of diagnosis, or the improvements since then.

The subjects of these first six chapters are all common sense. Whatever our health problems are; we all should regularly take a good honest look at ourselves and examine all of our actions and activities, to ascertain if any of them could be harmful. I have tried not to be too idealistic. All of us have some bad habits.

Because I do a lot of exercise, and am very active, my appetite is very good, with the result that I probably eat too much. I also continue to drink a sensible amount of alcohol, even though I know it is claimed not to be good for Pd. We do know that red wine and whisky have many health benefits. However, most people agree that we should limit our intake.

Eventually, in 2005, I found a medication, which is non-addictive and does not cease to be effective, after a period of time. My neurologist put me onto Trepiline, which I understand is not a sleeping pill but a tranquilizer, normally prescribed for Alzheimer's patients.

Scientists are fairly certain that Pd is caused by a combination of genetic and environmental factors, but I did not know this at the time of being diagnosed. This did not help me in my search for possible contributory factors, which could have brought on this terrible affliction. I did know that I was not leading a healthy lifestyle. I also knew that my attitude had become very negative and needed a good shake-up. But, other than these two facts, I found it rather difficult to put into words, all the collective thoughts and actions, which took place over those years. I have dealt with each aspect of my life, which had consciously been changed, in order to help me cope with the effects of the Pd.

I don't want the book to sound like a lecture. I want you to know that I have made many mistakes during this period, mainly by over-exercising. However, had I been a scholar, and read up everything about this disease, when I was diagnosed, I might conceivably have become completely discouraged, long before I experienced the first sign of Improvement.

You may wonder about the title of the seventh chapter, which deals with a very important personal discovery, which has changed my whole life. 'The final piece of the puzzle', is not something new to medical science, but something which, when applied to our movement disorder, and combined with all the other steps discussed in the first six chapters, completes the whole picture.

Chapter 1

Bodily Fitness

During my lifetime, I have unwittingly witnessed a major change in the lifestyle of urban communities throughout the Western world. Neither my father, nor any of his peers, would ever have dreamed of going to the gym, for an hour each day, before going to work. Yet, I, and many of my peers, would not dream of missing more than a day, without doing some form of exercise. This change in attitude has spawned the phenomenal growth of the health and fitness industry. This has taken several different directions, one of which has been the appearance of health clubs and gymnasiums, mainly in large urban areas. They have become firmly entrenched as part of the Western lifestyle. These facilities have always been available, since the beginning of the twentieth century, albeit, only for the privileged few.

Why the need for these facilities now?

We must all be aware that mechanization, in mining, farming and industry, has largely done away with the need for manual labor in the workplace. Simultaneous to this change, there has been a huge growth in the more sedentary occupations, and Service Industries. In addition to these changes, we have also experienced the proliferation of the motorcar, and other forms of public transport. So, instead of getting our daily exercise, by walking or cycling to work, and/or doing manual labor in the workplace, we now have to get our daily exercise by running, jogging, walking, swimming or working-out in the gym. There is, of course, the other option of taking part in some kind of regular sporting activity, but this is difficult to do on a daily basis. This assumes that we are all health conscious and want to stay reasonably healthy.

The problem is, because exercise is not forced upon us any more, as it was in the past, only the more motivated people among us actually get enough.

There are far too many other titillating alternatives to physical exercise, available at our fingertips, to while away our spare time and eat up our scarce financial resources. Unfortunately, taking part in healthy activities requires a fair amount of physical effort, which does not necessarily make it all that popular.

On the whole, we have also become spectators, rather than participants, in general sporting activities. Add to this, the time many of us spend commuting back and forth to work, and we get a fair picture of a potentially unhealthy situation.

If you are one of those unfortunate people, who have been struck down by Pd, then you need to take a really good look at your present situation.

Be brutally honest with yourself!

If you have neglected your bodily fitness in the past, then you will probably experience a certain reluctance to suddenly embark upon a fitness program. Unfortunately, I believe this is the **only** way that you will be able to improve your physical and mental fitness, and thereby, your own quality of life. Don't think that because you are currently unable to walk very fast, or very far, that you cannot possibly think of embarking on an exercise program. **You CAN!** Most people can, regardless of their state of health. Even bedridden people can do some form of exercise. You must expect to start at your present level of fitness, whatever that is, and build up **SLOWLY,** to the required level. As you build up, you will immediately feel the benefit of doing that exercise, and the further you progress, the greater will be the benefits. Whatever you choose to do as exercise, be it walking, running, swimming, exercising in a gym or horse-riding, that is your choice. No exercise is a waste of time or energy. Some exercises are better for Pd than others.

Mental fitness is just as important as physical fitness. The brain uses a great deal of energy, and using it to do difficult tasks affects it very positively. You may think that you are no good at puzzles or playing bridge or, any other form of mental exercise. Fair enough! If you have never done anything like this before, then set your mind to learning, from the very beginning. People do not look down on beginners; in fact they normally go out of their way to encourage them. You will derive a great deal of pleasure from learning new skills, and taking part in playing card games with other people. Try not to get too serious about any of these exercises, it could make you more stressed, and you don't need that. Play for fun and entertainment; the benefits derived from taking part will be a bonus. What you don't use, you lose! The brain is your most important organ, and it is at the root of the problem, so the more you use it, the better it will be.

Taking medication should **not be the only** remedial action we take, when we are faced with a serious health problem. We should never abdicate the responsibility of control over our own lives to other people. We should never rely on medication alone to restore or balance our state of health. In our case, **medication is a necessity**, but we should continually examine our daily lifestyle. Then set about taking steps to try to get rid of the bad habits and develop some good ones. If you have reached the stage where exercise is not an option, then I ask you to excuse me for making that assumption.

The golden rule in life is,

If you don't use it, you lose it!

This applies equally to all bodily functions, and any muscle, which is not used regularly, will naturally start to atrophy, **within seven days**. You cannot expect to have a healthy mind, if you don't have a healthy body. However, an injured, or partially mutilated, body can still remain healthy.

LOOK AFTER YOUR BODY, IT IS THE ONLY ONE YOU WILL EVER HAVE.

My current exercise routine consists of two visits a week to the 'Senior Citizen's Fitness Association' gym classes, where we do very important movement routines, to music, requiring a lot of mind-body coordination. We also do stretching and strengthening exercises. These are the three groups mentioned in **John Argue's**[2] presentation. I also do aerobic walking, normally three times a week, for eight kilometers (five miles) each time. This makes a total of twenty-four kilometers a week (fifteen miles). This may seem impossible to achieve for many people, but I didn't start at that level, I started at twenty minutes a session, during which I was only able to walk less than two kilometers (Just over a mile) to start with. As I progressed, I slowly built up the time by five minutes every second week, until I reached seventy minutes. I chose that amount of time because I chose, at that time, to walk ten kilometers a session.

---

[2] *Refer to the 3rd Presentation at the 1st World Parkinson's Conference, in Appendix 3.*

I must emphasize that I was not able to walk very well, when I embarked upon this Run/walk for Life program. I did not look forward to doing it, but I did it to prove to Shirley that it **would not help me**, because I had been doing far more exercise than just the walking, and my condition had continued to deteriorate. **How could I have been more wrong?**

Since picking up an injury in 2008, I have only been able to walk much shorter distances. In addition to that injury, I have been plagued by more back related problems, which have also curtailed my exercise program.

Money can buy most things, but it cannot buy good health. When ill-health strikes, there are few among us, who would not pay a lot of money to quickly get back the health we once had. If only we could take out an **insurance policy**, which would restore our health, not our wealth, when we suddenly get struck down with something like Pd, or when old age eventually catches up with us. Well, there is such an insurance policy, but the premiums cannot be paid in cash. **They have to be paid in physical effort.**

Maintaining your bodily fitness is the only insurance policy your body has, when ill health or old-age eventually catches up with you. You will then realize that all your efforts to maintain bodily fitness were as good as having put money into a bank, for that unexpected rainy day.

There is one advantage that your health problems generally have over your financial problems, usually associated with the loss of, or damage to, your possessions. On the one hand, when you get robbed, or break something, you can claim your money back from your insurance company. But, if you have not been paying your premiums, or weren't insured properly in the first place, you have a problem. On the other hand, if in the past, when life was treating you well, you had not been looking after your body, it is never too late to rectify that situation, even after ill health has struck. You can still embark upon a healthy exercise program, and get back into the habit of eating sensibly. At worst, you could stand a good chance of at least partially restoring your health to its former level. At best, you could fully recover, and continue to enjoy your life to the full. This assumes that you survived the health problem.

Ask any surgeon about the difference between operating on a bodily fit patient and someone who is unfit. He/she will tell you that, not only is it easier to perform an operation on someone who is fit, but the fit patient's chances of survival are far greater, and the recovery period is normally far shorter.

To give an example of this, my most recent back operation, which was occasioned by the damage done to my lower spine by my bad walking posture, involved more than five hours in the operating theatre. Although I was over sixty-five years of age, I had, at that time, been walking an average of more than thirty kilometers a week. I had the operation on a Wednesday afternoon, and came out of the theatre at about seven o'clock that first evening. The first morning after the operation, I asked the surgeon if he would have the catheter and drip removed, so that I could get up, which he arranged. With difficulty, I managed to get up and walk around the hospital for a total of more than an hour, that evening. On the second morning, following the operation, I managed to walk around the hospital corridors for more than three hours, altogether. When I saw the surgeon, that evening, and told him what I had managed to achieve during the day, I asked if I could go home the next morning, and he agreed. Before lunch on the Saturday, Shirley and I walked one and a half kilometers, around our suburb and, after taking a rest we walked another one and a half kilometers in the late afternoon. The next day we repeated the same distance in two separate walks, and from there on, we walked two kilometers each morning and afternoon. By the following Saturday, when I went to have my stitches removed, Shirley and I had managed to walk twenty-six kilometers (fifteen miles) together. This may seem like a bit of a tall story, I know, but it is absolutely true.

The most difficult problem, immediately after having an operation of this kind, is getting in and out of bed. If you have had a serious operation you will know what you go through, when getting out of bed. To do so, you have to grit your teeth, and just go for it. Initially, it feels as if the wound has split wide open and all the stitches have broken, but once on your feet, the pain level becomes quite bearable. After a while, you forget that it is even there. My wound healed incredibly quickly, due, I am told, to the increased blood flow to the wound, which was brought about by the regular raised levels of exertion over prolonged periods of time.

We all have to have a reason to get out of bed in the morning, other than needing to go to the bathroom. We must have a purpose to our lives. It is said that *we all need to be needed,* but this is not always possible. However, what better purpose can there be than the need to take care of our own health? It is our duty to ourselves, and our families to do this; otherwise we could become **a burden to them**.

The mere thought of becoming completely dependent upon other people, to wash and dress ourselves, is enough to motivate the most reluctant sufferers, to give it their best shot.

So, it is not surprising that Pd is not an easy problem for many sufferers to manage. It is also not surprising that sufferers often become very negative about their general prognosis. I am painfully aware that;

ONLY *WE* CAN HELP OURSELVES.

Others can help us to help ourselves, but nobody else can do exercise for us, or keep our minds active.

We cannot criticize fellow PwPs, who choose to give in to Pd, and throw in the towel, especially if they feel that they have reached the end of their useful lives. It is very difficult to motivate people who have made this choice. It is not anybody else's business to intervene in this situation, providing the patient's decision has not been made in ignorance.

In my opinion, my good fortune has come to me in four different ways, which I am certain has helped me to get to where I am now.

- I have a very supportive wife and family.
- I have been compelled to do a fair amount of exercise over the years, because of my back problems. Bodily, I was very fit **when diagnosed**.
- I managed to give up my job, without too much financial strain being placed upon my family.
- My neurologist prescribed a monotherapy of the only medication that can slow down, or even reverse the progress of Pd..

My back problem, as painful as it has been, paid me a big dividend, later in life, for which I am very grateful. Had I not taken part in that musical, back in 1961, and lifted the leading lady up in the air, my 'improved condition' may never have happened.

At the time of diagnosis, I had been going to gym and running for a number of years, as recommended to me by my chiropractor, because of the state of my health at that time. As I have already said, I am not very fond of exercise or sport and, to begin with, I was very reluctant to put so much effort into doing something, which was very painful and I didn't enjoy.

Before I had the first disc removed in 1977, at the age of forty-three, I had started jogging on a regular basis. I had got to the point, after a year or two, where I was running as much as fifteen kilometers (Nine Miles), without any problem and, being happy with that distance, had no ambition to go any further. I had no desire to enter for marathons, as I really did not have the time. This situation continued until the mid-eighties, when I started to develop a knee problem, which was then diagnosed as osteoarthritis, but was later traced back to the newly acquired habit of supinating[3], while running. Consequently, I found it too painful to run, and reluctantly decided to only exercise at the gym instead.

I did still play the odd game of golf, but that was no more than once a year. The last time I played golf, was at Sun City, in 1989, when the company took all my staff and their partners for a long weekend, close to Christmastime. I was teamed up with the Managing Director and Sales Director of the company, who were both reasonably good players, (it's funny that they had the time to play golf regularly, when I didn't). After an hour and a half on that beautiful course, which was designed by Gary Player, I had lost five balls, and had only completed three holes. Had I been anybody else, the other two would have told me where to get off. They very kindly helped me look for my ball each time and made light of a tricky situation. The course is very taxing for a hacker like me, and I could not even manage to get from the tees onto any of the fairways, because there is a lot of rough between those two points. When I say rough, I really do mean *rough,* and nobody wants to get lost, without a gun, in that stuff.

The cause of my problem was my bad muscle co-ordination. I could not hit that ball in any manner that could vaguely be described as controlled. When I finished that third hole I told

---

[3]**Supinating** *is the action of walking, while favoring the outside of the foot. This is generally associated with Dystonia.* **Pronating** *is the action of walking, while favoring the inside of the foot.*

the others that, if we wanted to get finished before dark, I was prepared to concede the game and drop my ball onto the fairway, for three shots, and then play from there and chip it onto the green. I never played again after that.

By the end of 1992, I was walking at six kilometers per hour, for those twenty minutes on the treadmill, cycling at around fifteen kilometers per hour and climbing two-thousand steps, which is one hundred steps a minute. You may think that, at my age, I should have been satisfied with those results, but they were at least 20% less than I had been achieving six months previously.

After the aerobic exercises, I then went onto six different exercise machines, to do a series of three sets of ten (30) exercises at various fitness levels, using a variety of weights. Here again, the weight levels had come down quite noticeably over the previous six months, with no apparent reason, other than possibly the Pd.

Just before the diagnosis, I felt exhausted, long before the exercise regimen was completed, which had never happened to me before. Although I had always tried to do as much as I could, I felt that I had never consciously tried to do too much. Until six months before then, I had always felt good, after having my shower, and had in fact looked forward to going to the gym every day. My enjoyment might have had something to do with those very attractive leotards and the equally attractive young ladies who wore them!

At that time, I had assumed that I was falling asleep at work, because of the exhaustion, which I was experiencing after gym, and that was the main reason why I was seeing the neurologist. Because my GP had noticed my bad walking gait, he advised me to first go to a physician for a general check-up. When I entered this man's office, he told me to go back outside and come back in again. This astounded me! He happened to have noticed, when I walked into his office that I was not walking very well and, in fact, much worse than I had on my visit to him twelve months before. After a thorough examination, he recommended that I visit a neurologist, as he was not happy about my walking and my overall condition.

After the Pd diagnosis, I carried on at the gym for another two years, during that period of 'mourning", while I watched my performance gradually deteriorating. This was truly soul-destroying for me, even though I knew that I had the Pd, and had been warned to expect a gradual decline in my overall condition, I never expected it to deteriorate so quickly. I also noticed that I was getting progressively clumsier in my movements. It is hard to be specific about this. For example: even while in the gym, I became very unsure of myself, walking between the machines, often bumping into pieces of equipment and other people. I felt that this was because there was nothing to hold onto, not realizing that I should not need something to support me. In fact, I sometimes acted as though I had had a little too much to drink. I used to go to the gym at six o'clock in the morning, because that was when they opened and, while I was still working, was the only available time I could find for this very important part of my daily life.

While all of this was happening, Shirley had been taking part in 'Run/Walk for Life (RWFL)', which is a controlled walking or running program, since 1991. She did this mainly to lose weight, but also to get out of the house and away from the office. Shirley has never been one for exercise either, and the thought of walking several kilometers, three times a week, did not appeal to her at all. However, you can never accuse Shirl of a lack of determination. She set out to lose weight and by golly, she did exactly that! Shirley's blood pressure dropped to normal, during that time, after having taken blood-pressure pills for over twenty years. We had worked together in the business since its inception, and the stress affected her as much as it had me. She is a hardworking, dedicated person, who never gives up either. As I said before, my working hours affected her more than they did me.

When she told me how well she was doing and how well she was feeling, while my condition continued to go downhill; she suggested that I give it a try. I said, rather impatiently, that I was already walking for twenty minutes *every* day, plus a whole lot of other exercises, and what could walking on its own do for me? She kept up the low-level pressure on me, believing wholeheartedly that it would do me good, even though she was not sure why. Eventually, in 1994, I was so upset about my performance in the gym that I succumbed to the pressure and joined RWFL, feeling a bit negative but, what the hell, what did I have to lose?

The 'Walk for Life' program starts with ten minutes of warming-up and stretching exercises, designed to prevent anybody getting injured by damaging cold muscles, while doing strenuous exercise.

Beginners start off walking for ten minutes, around a school playing field. They are encouraged to increase their time by five minutes, every second week, until they can manage to walk a distance of four kilometers per session, when the member is then encouraged to walk on the road. The instructor keeps a record of distances and times, so that all the members have a complete record of their individual performances. When a member reaches his or her goal, then the instructor sets a new one, and so it goes, until they reach eight kilometers in distance per walking session.

Once a month, a time trial is organized, where each member, on the road, is timed over a four-kilometer course, and all of these times are recorded. The instructor encourages everyone to achieve a better time each month, and helps, where necessary. In this way, members manage to lose weight, reduce blood pressure, firm-up muscles, loosen limbs and joints and generally get a lot fitter, without picking up injuries, due to bad walking habits or over-enthusiasm.

At the end of each walk, members are encouraged to walk around the playing field, at least once, to cool-off. This also helps the body to adjust to a lower level of exertion, before stopping. Apparently, this is better than stopping suddenly, with the heart racing at full tilt.

Regardless of whether you have Pd or not, this is a good program for everybody and an **absolute must for PwP's**. I do not get commission for this apparent sales talk, but I have to give credit, where credit is due.

Getting back to walking; the RWFL instructor noticed that I was walking with my head facing down towards the ground. Although she knew that I had Pd, like many people, she knew nothing at all about the disease. She did not know that standing and walking, while leaning forward, is a common problem amongst PwPs. I was not aware of it myself either, at that stage. She kept shouting to me across the field to "Stand up straight, and look ahead", while I was walking. She made a point of getting me to pull my shoulders back and stand upright, thinking that I had developed this slouching position as a bad habit. Perhaps I had!

At the beginning, I was quite upset at only being allowed to walk for ten minutes, so she let me start at twenty minutes. Big deal! Walking on the field was rather uncomfortable for me; even though the surface was reasonably smooth, it is not possible to get a playing field absolutely flat, like a bowling green. I tripped and stumbled my way around that field for over two months, increasing my walking distance to four kilometers per session, before she would allow me onto the road. As a result of keeping a record of every single walk, I **was able to compare my times accurately**.

To my amazement, I not only found that I had increased my distance, which did not surprise me, but I had also significantly improved my times. **That was the first time my performance had improved in anything, for longer than I could remember.** You have no idea what affect that had on my mental state, at that time.

This was the turning point in the progress of my Parkinson's disease. The time I started to become positive about my future prospects.

Right from the beginning, the instructor did not give me any choice. I had to walk at each level, for at least two weeks, before she would let me increase my distance by a further kilometer, each time. Eight weeks after I got onto the road, I reached my set goal of eight kilometers. From memory, my times were then around eight and a half minutes per kilometer. I have to admit that one or two of the ladies beat me, hands down, on all distances, and they trounced me on the monthly time trials as well. Fortunately, I don't think I have too much of a male ego problem, and even if I had, there was no way in which I could have beaten them!

The quality of my walking action was, unbeknown to me, rather clumsy. Only when I entered into a ten-kilometer family walk, did somebody complain that I was running, and not walking. When I spoke to my instructor, after the walk, she agreed that it did indeed look as if I was running, but she understood the problem and had tried to persuade the judges that I was, in fact, walking and, because of my Pd, was unable to walk normally. Bearing in mind that I had only come in fifth overall, and as the ten-kilometer walk was only a fun walk, they did nothing about it. I talked to my instructor about the problem again, after that race, and she promised to help me. But, try as we may, we could not get my legs to come down with a straight knee, when the heel touched the ground, as it should, when walking properly. As this did not worry anybody in our RWFL group, even on the time trials, I did not pay too much attention to the problem, and just got on with improving my times. I managed to get down to six and three quarter minutes per kilometer, over the full eight-kilometer course, with which I was very pleased. This superb time, for me, was still not good enough to better some of those, not so young ladies, who were always willing to help me do better.

Shirley lost fourteen kilograms in her first year, and managed to maintain her weight for eight years after that, until she had to give up the walking, because of osteoarthritis in her knees and feet. She had to start taking the blood pressure pills again, two years after ceasing the 'Walk for Life" program. She is still hoping to get back to her walking. I managed to lose a few kilograms as well, but as that was not one of my goals, I don't remember exactly how many.

We continued with RWFL until 1998 when, due to the instructor's retirement, we had to move to another group, which was situated a further six kilometers away from where we lived. Unfortunately for us, this took close on an extra half hour to reach in the rush-hour traffic, and we soon lost heart and decided to walk on our own, around our own suburb. We had been doing the aerobic walking for such a long time that we didn't need any incentive to get up in the morning. I was very pleased, at the time, because I was under the mistaken impression that by walking every day, I would then be able to get a lot fitter than I had been, while walking only three times a week. We were very grateful to the RWFL people for the part they had played in improving our joint health and, had it not been for them, I think that I would still be going to gym and would probably have given up long ago.

Many months later, my back problem returned, with the result that I had to stop walking for some time. This was all caused by exercising too much, and the fact that I was walking in a bent forward position, which put a lot of pressure on the lower back and ruptured another disc. That put an end to walking more than three times a week.

The improvement in my condition had been so gradual, that it was impossible to monitor in any way. What happened in practice was that I would suddenly realize that one or other of my symptoms had either got a lot better, without my having noticed, or had disappeared altogether. For non-PwPs, this may sound a bit difficult to understand but, like many other injuries, which happen to us during our lives, we quickly learn to adjust to the new situation. When we get accustomed to the tremor, it becomes part of our daily life. We can adjust to anything, as we do with spectacles and false teeth.

The first change, which came to my attention, was my facial appearance. Friends and acquaintances regularly stopped me in the mall, or in one of my erstwhile factories, when I visited, and told me how well I was looking. This seemed to me at first to be a kindly gesture on their part, meant to cheer me up. My health had slowly been deteriorating for such a long time that family and friends alike had got used to thinking of me as an 'invalid'. So, this improvement had become very noticeable to those who did not see me very often, but had not really been noticed by my family. But, when they thought about it, they realized that there had been a very noticeable change in my general health. I also started to realize that I was a lot more cheerful, and had more confidence. I was physically able to smile again.

When these friends and acquaintances told me that I was looking a lot better, I sometimes got the distinct impression that many of them thought I must have purposely misled them, because the one thing that everybody knows about Pd is that it is incurable. This feeling, of being suspected of putting on an act, has not worried me unduly, although it has been a bit hurtful. I know that I could be imagining their reactions to seeing me, but I don't think so. The facts speak for themselves, and those who are close to me, know exactly what I have been through.

What suddenly dawned on me was that, after I had received that initial diagnosis, I had conditioned my mind to the fact that *I could never get better*. I believed I could only get worse.

That was a very negative attitude.

This was a very important realization. How can we expect to get better, or even start to feel better, if we have conditioned our minds to believe that *we can only get worse?* This negative attitude tends to become a self-fulfilling prophecy.

Upon reflection, the improvement, in my overall performance, might have had something to do with the fact that, since I gave up the gym in 1994, I was only exercising for about an hour every second day, as against the one and a half hours every single day, which I had been doing in the gym previously. I was no longer getting tired either, and I was beginning to feel quite perky, for the first time in many years.

You can imagine that, when my health had been going downhill at a rate I could actually notice, what a joy it was to witness a genuine improvement in my performance at anything physical.

I have not been involved in any organized sport, since my twenties (mainly squash), although I did try to play regular golf, after I first got married, but time constraints soon put a stop to that. So, don't conjure up any picture of a super-fit athlete, trying to persuade a few dedicated couch potatoes to become enthusiastic about physical exercise. By nature, I'm with the couch potatoes, but circumstances have forced me to become a fitness freak, and to take full control of my own destiny.

When I think back on it, I often wonder what would have happened, had I not been doing all that exercise. I have heard an eminent neurologist, in South Africa say at an 'Information Day', "Exercise makes no difference at all to the progression of Pd". I am personally convinced that, contrary to his thinking, it has had a great deal to do with *my* present state of health. I now know that is absolute nonsense. I have read many articles this past few years, written by leading neurologists throughout the world, stating that exercise *has* a very important part to play in slowing down the progression of Pd. Speaking now, whilst writing the second re-write of the book, we know for certain that exercise has a very definite affect on the brain and the body. More of that later!

So much has happened in Parkinson's circles, over the past eight years, since writing the first book, that I am now in the position to say emphatically that the **two major points I have made about, what we should all be doing to ward off the inevitable progression of Pd, have been proven to be absolutely correct.**

I have been receiving regular journals/newsletters from various Parkinson's organizations around the world for a number of years, including SPRING Times and Northwest Parkinson's Foundation Post. Up until recently, these media were almost entirely filled with news about new medications, surgery and various other forms of medical treatment. However, over the past three or four years, this situation has suddenly started to change, and they now give more information on what we can all do for ourselves, in the way of exercise and alternative therapies[4].

Many of my readers will be very doubtful about their own ability to start doing such strenuous exercise. I want to remind you that exercise sessions should start with warm-up exercises, for several minutes. These warm-up exercises are not strenuous and would be what **you are capable of doing.** You would not be expected to do anything more than you are capable of. The warm-up exercises would be followed by the walking, at your pace, for as little as **a few minutes**. From There it can build up by doing a little more every second week, until you have reached the goal of one hour, three times a week. Most of us are still able to perform *some* movement, under proper supervision, and we can all build on that, while our bodies will do the rest. As we get better at the exercise, we will find we will start to realize we are feeling better, and that realization will give us the will to go further. **It was that realization, after three months of walking seriously, that my condition *was* starting to improve, which gave me the determination to continue walking.** You have no idea how motivating that was.

All the exercise I have done, plus everything I have read about the affect of exercise on the progression of Pd, indicates to me that there is a proven benefit to the brain from doing regular energetic exercise. There is also a benefit to be derived from keeping the brain active. The older people living in our retirement village, who keep active, are far healthier than those who just sit and watch television. Many of them are in their nineties and still play bridge. One old lady of ninety-five still plays Mah-Jong. This particular lady also does her own gardening, as do many others.

The details of the controlled study on exercise, leads me to believe that the restorative effect of GDNF (Glial Derived Neurotrophic Factor), produced in my brain, whilst running, and doing my gym exercises, during those years between 1964 and 1992, could well have been the reason for the slow progress of my Pd, before I was diagnosed.

---

[4] *Refer to 'Alternative and Adjunctive Therapies' in Appendix 4.*

Chapter 2
Diet & Eating

After several years of trying to lose weight, by using this or that diet, I now believe in the simple axiom of,

'Moderation in everything, including moderation!'

Healthy eating is better than dieting. It has to be a way of life, not something you do for three weeks, before resuming your original **bad eating habits.**

Any diet, which is extreme, is not healthy in my opinion. Cutting out any food group, for whatever reason, does not make too much sense to me either. As we were created to be meat and vegetable eaters, our bodies are adequately equipped to handle both of these food groups, and we obviously need the vitamins and nutrients that we get from both sources. In our more primitive past, there would not always have been the opportunity to eat a balanced diet, due to the non-availability of certain food items at all times. Therefore, the chances are that our bodies are also capable of handling an unbalanced diet on a daily basis, provided that we eat a balanced diet over a period of time.

We have learned that PwP's must be careful with certain food types, specifically proteins, because of a conflict with medication, and not the disease itself. I personally eat as little red meat as possible, sticking mainly to free-range chickens, pork and veal. Shirley and I eat a fair amount of fish and pasta. Our pasta meals, generally, do not include meat, but do often include various seafood items.

My reluctance to eat much red meat emanates from a serious problem I had in the past, which concerned my Eldepryl tablets. On that occasion, I suffered from a blocked bowel, after foolishly going onto a high protein diet, with Shirley. As mentioned earlier, we both have a bit of a weight problem, and for years we tried to find a diet that suited us, but to no avail. I am sure that more than half the Western world has been on one diet or another, during the past thirty years, but invariably, they all revert back to their original weight, after coming off the diet. Some people we know have even exceeded their original weight, after coming off a diet.

The one substance that I try not to take in any form is caffeine, because I observed that, after drinking a lot of coffee,

52

my tremors were definitely more pronounced, and after cutting out coffee and tea altogether, my hand tremors slowly disappeared. This may have been a coincidence, because it happened at the same time as I learned to **bypass my subconscious brain,** see Part 4. I have seen in the press that caffeine is capable of protecting us from Pd, but that is a bit late for me. One day I might experiment with drinking coffee again, but I don't feel any need at present to do so, and I am sure that water is a lot healthier than either tea or coffee. I still occasionally drink wine, even though it is recommended that PwPs don't. But, because it positively affects my blood pressure, and because I like it, I drink it in moderation, and by no means every day.

We should all give a wide berth to the widely used chemical, Aspartame, which occurs in many food and drinks products. It has 92 serious neurological side effects, which can be seen on the internet. You should check on the labels of all the products you consume, to see if it appears. It has been known to have very detrimental neurological and other effects on certain patients. Be aware of it.

About 10 years ago, it was found that grapefruit juice interacts with some blood pressure and other medications. It has turned out that grapefruit juice, uniquely among other citrus drinks, increases the bioavailability of several medications. The cause of this is the effect of the juice on an enzymatic system in the liver, which metabolize medication. The most important effects are on the drugs Cyclosporin, calcium-antagonist antihypertensive medications, and various statin agents. Some Valium derivatives, carbamazepine, Zoloft, as well as other medications are also affected. These interactions are significant and should be discussed with your treating doctor or patients should simply avoid grapefruit juice altogether[5].

If you take Azilect or Eldepryl, you should be aware that **you should avoid any food that contains tyramine,** the breakdown of which is inhibited by the medication. When tyramine builds up in the body, it can cause extremely high blood pressure. **Hence my high blood pressure problems[6].** Consult your dietician to find out what foods contain tyramine, or Google "Tyramine" on the internet.

---

[5] *Mayo Clinic Proceedings, 2000*
[6] *Refer to Chapter 4, Medication*

Other than these three changes in my diet, I find it difficult to swallow dry substances, like potatoes and bread and even dry, well-done, meat. I have to eat these food items with something moist, or with a nice sauce.

As I don't drink tea or coffee any more, I prefer to drink filtered tap water. This may sound terribly boring to lots of people, but it is more refreshing than any gassy cool drink (Soda). The problem is that it is not considered very sociable to visit someone and ask for a glass of tap water, while everybody else is having a hot cup of tea or coffee. What can I say? Social norms have developed over the centuries and will not change in a day, simply because I have Pd, and don't want to have any caffeine. Besides, if I tell people that I have Pd, they look at me as if I am pulling a fast one, so it is easier to say that I simply prefer water to anything else, and leave it at that. Our son has never drunk tea or coffee in his life. He also prefers water.

I have also tried taking vitamins and have come to the conclusion that, in my case, they are expensive and unnecessary, providing that I eat a balanced diet. I experienced no noticeable benefits whatsoever, after taking multi-vitamins for a period of several months. So, why bother to take them? Again, I am sticking my neck out, and will definitely get it chopped off by many of my readers, but there it is! I have not heard any dietician say we must or must not take dietary supplements, so I assume that eating lots of fruit and vegetables gives us all the vitamins we need.

A lot is said about anti-oxidants these days. I do agree with the beneficial effects they might have on our health, and the possible need to have a good intake of them on a daily basis. As I have said, I eat a very healthy diet, with lots of fresh vegetables and fruit. I have never taken any anti-oxidant supplements, other than garlic pills, but am considering doing so. There is no proof that these anti-oxidants get through the blood-brain barrier, so they may not actually help us. I feel that a controlled double-blind study should be done on this subject.

There are two supplements, which I do take for health reasons. The first, I have mentioned, is three garlic capsules, which are an anti-oxidant, every day; as I have done since before I was diagnosed. I used to chop up a clove of garlic into small pieces and wash them down with a glass of tap water. For those of you, who cringe at the thought of bad breath, let me say that this seems not to have been a problem, as long as I didn't chew the garlic. However, there was initially a little flatulence during the first week or so, after which, even that disappeared. I also take one chelated calcium and magnesium tablet per day. They apparently are the best. I believe this to be necessary, bearing in mind that I have a lactose intolerance problem, from time to time, and I don't drink any milk or eat much cheese with a high fat content. I have no medical training but I do know that there is a problem getting calcium into the blood stream. It apparently needs to piggyback onto another chemical, in order to get through. Taking any old calcium tablets does not guarantee that you get the benefit of the calcium, where you need it.

It must be borne in mind that I do not take any medication containing Levodopa. I mention this because if you are taking Levodopa medication, you should be aware that **other foodstuffs compete for the Levodopa in the gut,** and if you have certain foodstuffs containing protein in your gut, when you take your medication, you will get less Levodopa into the brain, which is where it is needed. It is generally felt that you should take your medication at least three-quarters of an hour, or even an hour, **before** you eat anything with protein in it. If you are unable to wait that time in the morning, before breakfast, then avoid protein. You should also not take medication for at least the same period of time **after** eating. It varies from person to person, and it could be more than an hour for some.

If you do find that you have been eating protein within the times mentioned above, and you decide to change that situation, you might find that you get too much dopamine in your brain, which could cause you problems. This can be rectified by taking less medication, but first speak to your doctor.

Chapter 3

Stress Management

Rest and relaxation were not the only benefits I derived from giving up my job. Without realizing it, when I gave up my career at the end of 1992, I had succeeded in:

Removing most of the issues that caused me to be negatively stressed.

I am aware that none of us can survive without a certain level of stress, and do not believe that it is possible to have no stress whatsoever. Without going *too* deeply into the subject, which would be a book all on its own, I would just like to emphasize that we all *need* a certain level of stress in our daily lives. But we can all do without the type of *negative stress* that makes the blood pressure rise to unhealthy levels, keeping us awake at night and giving our collective GP's anxiety attacks. That is the type of stress that I left behind, when I stopped working.

In 1974, I attended a very short 'Seminar' on retirement planning, which was really an excuse to sell insurance. The only thing that I remember about that 'Seminar' was something we should all take note of, every day of our working lives. We were strongly advised not to enter our retirement, **without a definite plan** of what we intended doing with our newfound freedom. There is nothing more likely to bring about our demise than suddenly finding that we have nothing to do. Good advice! There is nothing worse for a man, than having nothing to do, and all day in which to do it. Women do not generally have the same problem, as they always have something to do. We men see to that!

There was no such plan in my mind, when I suddenly decided to retire. I was unable to participate any more in golf or bowls. I am not a social drinker and had no circle of friends in a position to keep me company, during those long daylight hours ahead of me. I did not belong to any clubs, where businessmen often entertain their friends and business acquaintances. In fact, I had no close circle of friends I could latch onto, for enjoying shared activities.

The very activity that caused most of the negative stress in the first place, came to my rescue. Yes, **my computer** was my savior. It gave me an avenue to occupy my time, without causing me any stress, related to deadlines or performance. I had the time to clean up those programs, and put in features that I never had time to do in the past. It became some sort of catharsis. I was able to polish up the programs and pass them on to my company, and my customers, and put my mind at rest. In the back of my mind, I felt that I had previously failed, both in my job, as head of my company, and in my determination to create the perfect programs to run my business. How many of us have been satisfied at the end of our working lives that we have achieved everything we set out to do? This time-consuming job, on the computer, took nearly four years, but it was worth every minute to me.

I have never ever sat down on my computer and played computer games. I don't, to the best of my knowledge, even have games on my computer. Many of my friends play card games on their computers, in their spare time. I don't seem to have any spare time. Don't ask me why. It does make me sound terribly boring.

Now, is as good a time as any, to examine the main causes of negative stress for us Pd sufferers!

The first, and most obvious, cause is money; or rather, the lack of it. The lack of money imposes a very heavy burden upon all involved. The person responsible for providing for the family unit will feel different emotions to those who are not in that position. Feelings, such as failure, inadequacy, helplessness, defeat, frustration, foundering and incompetence, can have terrible effects on people, especially breadwinners. If a sufferer is in this position, the combination of the lack of sufficient money to pay for the family's needs, and the onset of an incurable, debilitating disorder, can be lethal. If you are in this invidious position, then you should seek the help of a counselor and, together with other members of your family, seek a solution to your problems. Ask yourself, "If you were to die right now, would it help your family?" I'm sure the answer would be "no", but regardless of that, assuming that you are in a loving relationship and you would be missed very much by your family, then **worrying about your problem will not help anyone**. You have to **take action**. Get help from professionals. Don't leave it.

You should not wait until your condition gets to the situation where nothing can be done to help you.

The second most obvious cause is our inter-personal relationships, which can be very stressful, especially if we battle to speak properly. Non-sufferers sometimes struggle to deal with our neurological condition, due to their lack of knowledge and understanding of it. Even with understanding and empathy, communication with us can sometimes be very difficult. Often, people tend to steer well clear of us.

The majority of Pd sufferers are over fifty years of age, and at that age, even their children can cause them a great deal of stress. The world is currently going through a huge state of change. Unemployment has become a very worrying reality in the lives of many of us, and our children and grandchildren, who could be very seriously affected by the lack of job opportunities. This could be very stressful to us. We are told that we should not feel responsible for the situations, into which our children get themselves, but it is very difficult to sit back and watch them flounder. However, we must put things into their proper perspective. We are responsible for our own lives, and those who are totally dependent upon us. Although our responsibility to our children ends, when they reach maturity, it is difficult to simply turn our backs on them.

We have to make very difficult decisions sometimes, relating to our children's problems. We have to ask ourselves, "Are we able to help them, without causing major problems for ourselves?" If the answer is no, then we have to tell them. They have to accept that they are the responsible party, and they have to find the solution to their own problems. This is called **tough love,** and it is possible that you should have done it sooner. If no resolution is found, you will probably become even more ill, and even less able to solve their problems.

You may also find that your relationship with a friend or fellow worker has, in some instances, become strained. This may be very stressful to you, as you have to continue to live your life, and you may not be in the situation to give that person a wide berth. That person may also be feeling stressed with the relationship. In both cases, it is advisable to put your cards on the table and have a frank discussion with him/her and try and resolve the matter. If resolution cannot be found then you should agree to cease the friendship.

The third most obvious cause is the lack of something to do in our spare time, especially when we do not have any spare finance. There is a tendency amongst older people, to tell themselves that they **can't** do certain things, or that they are **too old** to learn. This is something, with which, we all have to come to terms, as we grow older. In reality, we are never too old to learn, but the fear of making a fool of ourselves, especially in front of our children, sometimes prevents us from trying to learn new skills. There is nothing foolish about making mistakes, especially within a learning environment. So, we should take courage from others, and try to learn something new, to help us fill those empty hours. When a person says, **"I can't"**, he/she is really saying, **"I don't know how"**. It stands to reason that, unless we have been taught something, we cannot be expected to be able to do it. We might think we know how, but until we actually try, we will never know whether we can. Be brave; take on something new, which may require a lot of reading or research, but that all takes time, of which we have plenty. Learn a new sport, or take up a new hobby, which will require some learning and skills training. You must get fun and pleasure out of whatever you take up, otherwise it is a waste of your time and energy.

A fourth cause is fortunately less common, but just as serious. It affects many older people who find themselves all alone. If you are all alone, and you have Pd, you are really in an unenviable situation. The stress that loneliness brings with it is almost impossible to deal with. You need to get hold of someone to help you find a place to live, where there are other people, probably as lonely as yourself. You have the opportunity to look at other people's problems, and then take an interest in them. This will take your mind off your own problems and give you a new purpose in life. We have to look outwards in this situation, not inwards.

There are many other causes of stress, but whatever causes you to be stressed, you would be well advised to take action and do something about it. Ascertain the cause of the stress, whatever it may be, and deal with it. If you are unable to handle it on your own, then get a counselor to advise you. Don't leave it simmering in your mind. It will cause you untold harm and it will strongly influence the progression of your Pd.

Having got rid of all my *negative stress* has definitely been a major factor in my 'apparent recovery' process. Since giving up my job, I have realized that each time I have allowed myself to become involved in projects and activities, which I allowed to get out of hand, I soon became stressed again.

To explain this in more detail, I must emphasize that not all of my activities, over the years since diagnosis, have caused me to become stressed, only those that changed from, being purely for pleasure, to being a total commitment. Some people *like* to get totally involved in projects, outside of the family and work situations, which are very time-consuming and fulfilling activities. But, these activities invariably require a complete commitment, from everyone involved.

The most notable example of this was my enrolment into my church choir. I was very busy at that time, re-writing some software, for my company but, seeing that I was going to church anyway, I decided that I might as well sing in the choir. At the beginning, I had to learn to read music, which you may find difficult to believe, bearing in mind how many years I have been singing. My eyesight is very poor and maybe, because of it, I have always been a very slow reader. I have worn thick glasses since I was seven years of age, not long after the Second World War began.

As a young child, I could not read what was on the blackboard and had to remember what the teacher had said. Even when I got my first pair of glasses, I found reading difficult. I only started reading for pleasure in my late twenties, up until which time, reading was really not a pleasure at all. I found that I had to concentrate so hard on the actual reading that I did not properly take in the content of what I was reading. I never ever read the lesson during a church service, for fear of making a fool of myself, due to mispronunciation and stumbling over difficult and confusing names.

I have seemingly deviated off the story about the church choir. I enjoyed being able to follow the music from the book, but could never do it fast enough to be able to read the music and the words at the same time. The organist, who was very professional, became quite frustrated with me, when I could not mouth the correct words, even if I happened by chance to have hit the correct note. She could read the music, play the organ, sing one of the parts and still listen to the choir singing. She never missed a wrong note or word, nor did she miss bad timing. In my mind, she was incredible, but her super ability made me feel very inadequate. I felt that I could never aspire to being able to maintain her standards. I was letting the rest of the choir down, by not being able to meet that standard.

Unfortunately for me, she was not in a position to understand my dilemma, nor was I able to explain it to her. Hence, I became very stressed, once more.

When I joined the choir, I had imagined that there would not be much extra work involved, but little did I realize that there were compulsory rehearsals and extra rehearsals for special functions, at Christmas and Easter, not to mention the odd funeral or wedding and, of course, all the extra travelling.

Slowly, the overall workload exceeded the available time, and the obligation to have to excuse myself from practices at short notice, when I really did not need the extra work in the first place, soon found me in a no-win situation. I was struggling with the music, I was struggling to fulfill all of my obligations to my family and my company, and one day, when the proverbial brown stuff hit the fan, something snapped, and I, uncharacteristically, threw in the towel.

I am telling you this, not to get it off my chest, but to illustrate the type of activity that has given me that *negative stress*. Life has been difficult enough, without having had to commit myself to other activities, which put enormous demands on my non-existent spare time.

There comes a time in life when something has to give. Sometimes, we leave it too late and our minds and/or bodies give in under the strain. Afterwards, we ask ourselves, "Was it really worth it?" The answer, in my case was 'No!' My job and my family put enough demands on me for one lifetime, and all other commitments were incidental. There have been other occasions, since my diagnosis, when I became unreasonably stressed. Each time this happened, some of the more noticeable symptoms slowly returned again, even while I was still on the Eldepryl tablets. In each instance, my family or I suddenly became more aware of the Pd. Luckily, in every instance, my condition soon returned to normal, after getting rid of the stress.

Now, I fill my spare time with painting and sculpting. I am taking art lessons once a week and am enjoying them immensely. Art has been of interest to me, in the past, not so much as an admirer but as a participant. When my children were at school, I took great pleasure in helping them with their homework projects, just to make them aware of what they could achieve themselves, without cutting pictures out of good books or magazines. Over the years, I have learned to paint and sculpt to a fairly acceptable level. The satisfaction derived from the hours spent putting paint onto canvas or paper, is immeasurable, and the pleasure I have shared with my fellow budding artists, has been a welcomed bonus. My first art teacher was amazed at the improvement in my hand tremor, since I started learning. In 1999, when I first went to the zoo, with fellow students, I was not able to sketch the animals properly, because the lines were so shaky. The harder I tried to draw a straight line, the more my hand shook. However, I am a very determined person, and I was not going to be beaten by this impediment. So, by concentrating hard on what I was doing, I somehow found a way to overcome this problem, and can now draw lines without any of those tell-tale squiggles.

When I was down in Port Elizabeth, for the Annual General Meeting of the Parkinson Association (PASA), on the 3rd of July 2001, I saw some lovely paintings of flowers, which had been lovingly painted by another PwP, and given to the Association, to help raise funds. So, I am not alone in having found art as a pastime, and I am sure that there are plenty of other PwPs out there, pursuing relaxing hobbies.

In the early months of 2010, I decided to make a CD, for my children and grandchildren, so that they had a verbal contact with me, after I have moved on to the next level. I am now taking singing lessons, for the first time in my life, and am going to finish the CD before Christmas.

For many years, the incredible achievements of women have fascinated me. I am not talking about physical attraction, although I am just as enamored of women as are most men.

The women I have in mind are the single mothers, who manage to hold down a job, bring up and care for a family, run a home and sometimes even maintain an active social life. This is still a fairly new phenomenon. When I was a young man, the concept, of an unmarried working mother, running a home and bringing up her children alone, would have been unthinkable. When I thought about this problem, I soon realized that an even larger number of women have been doing this for centuries. The only thing that has changed is that they now get paid for the work they do.

Why do I mention this in relation to Pd? The answer is related to the subject of 'Stress'. I would wager that most men would collapse under the stress of having to look after their children, clean a house, cook the food, buy the family essentials, keep a job and earn enough money to pay for the family's needs. Add to this, the task of looking after a demanding partner and you have an idea of why I would take this wager. There are few men around who could handle that level of stress.

I have become aware, in my later years, that women are seemingly able to ignore adversity, when it comes to looking after children and husbands. Women can be dying on their feet, but the urge to look after others, enables them to carry on, when a large number of us men would have already given up long ago. I never cease to be amazed by what women can achieve, under difficult circumstances. I think that, generally, women tend to be more organized and focused than men.

It is not possible to talk to everybody at the meetings I attend, but I keep my eyes and ears open, and ask the ladies and the men, or their helpers, various questions relating to their daily routines, and what they do to overcome their problems. Meetings are a good place to gather information, and the more we learn about the disease, the better we will be equipped to deal with it on a daily basis.

I have not carried out any scientific study of the women sufferers I have met, over the past few years, but I have formed a very clear image in my mind of, amongst other things, the differences I have noticed in the progression of the disease, among the majority of those women sufferers. This differs greatly from the progression of the disease, amongst the majority of male sufferers, whom I have met.

It is wrong to generalize, but it has been quite plain to me, for many years now that men generally do not cope with Pd as well as women do. They seem to go downhill much quicker than the ladies, with a few notable exceptions, and the reason appears to be rather obvious. Men don't normally have homes to run, meals to cook and grandchildren to look after. This is said with my tongue in my cheek, but you all know what I mean. We old men have been spoilt rotten all our lives, by those wonderful women we were lucky to have married, and we have had many years to develop the habit of leaving all these tasks to our wives. This realization might be counter to the fact that women lead more stressful lives than men, therefore, if I am right about stress being counter-productive, then women should go downhill faster than men. I think that the workload that many women tend to bear is not necessarily as stressful to them as it would be to us men.

Shirley seldom went to bed, when she did not feel too good. She never watched TV after work, because she had to get the dinner ready. This sounds like a lot of woman talk, but it was true. I have worked very hard all my life, and I did enjoy it as much as Shirley enjoyed hers. The big difference was that I knew when my work was finished, and when I could relax, and play dominoes with my pal next door. Whereas, Shirley just carried on working until everything was finished. It never occurred to me to help her with 'her' work. When she had finished 'her chores', she usually picked up her knitting or crocheting and her hands were never idle. This seems to be what makes the difference.

Speaking to female PwPs I often asked them what they did at home, I generally found that they still cooked and did the housework, even though they took a lot longer than they used to. They were invariably still involved with grandchildren. These activities, and the exercise they derive from them, are probably the reasons why the Pd seems to progress slower in women than it does in men. I can hear the doctors saying "How can he make such wild statements, without doing proper research?" Well, they are quite right of course, I cannot prove what I have just said, and I cannot generalize on such a complex subject, because we are all different, and we all have our own specific problems, and cannot be compared to others. It is merely an observation. It is also a good subject for another controlled study.

My generation still had definite role models. Men did men's work and women did everything else. However, this is not the case today. The roles tend now to be shared by both sexes. Therefore, it will be interesting to see if the progression of Pd presents the same picture amongst the modern generation, as it has amongst mine. Their lives are more stressed than ours were at their age, which seems rather peculiar, when you consider all the gadgets they have to help them. If my feeling, that *negative* stress is a major contributor to the onset of Pd, is correct, then there should be an increase in the incidence of Pd now, especially amongst younger people.

Regardless of whether you have Pd or not, it is wise to avoid *negative* stress, wherever possible.

Chapter 4

Medication

For obvious reasons, I cannot pass comment about the advantages of one medication over another, because I am not qualified to do so. I have only had personal experience with Eldepryl for ten years and Sinamet for three months.

We all have the right to question and understand any medication our doctor prescribes. Ideally, doctors should explain to us what each of our medications does, and what its possible side effects are. They should also explain how long that medication will stay effective, and what else is available, when that medication ceases to be effective. There are certain types of medication, which have long-lasting effects on the central nervous system. It therefore stands to reason that these medications should only be prescribed, when no other less harmful medication is available to help us.

As I have said, I was very lucky indeed. My neurologist prescribed a monotherapy of Eldepryl (Selegiline), when he diagnosed the Pd. Since writing the first edition I have tried to establish whether many other people have been prescribed a monotherapy of an MAO-B inhibitor. Full details about MAO-B inhibitors appear in Appendix 4. None of the patients I have spoken to, up until 2010 have had this, and very few of them had even used an MAO-B inhibitor at all

Up until the beginning of January 2001, I took two tablets every day, other than on the odd occasions, when I forgot, and on three separate occasions, when I incorrectly thought I could manage without them. Many neurologists do not prescribe Eldepryl, or the latest MAO-B inhibitor – Azilect[7] - which is of a similar type. For some reason, they seem to overlook it, maybe because of one possible serious side effect, namely hypertension, which did seriously affect me. But, as a layman, I find it hard to understand why doctors do not first prescribe an MAO-B inhibitor. This is, to the best of my knowledge, the only group of drugs that have been proven to be able to slow down, or even reverse, the progression of Pd. Is it because they are just in the habit of prescribing other drugs?

---

[7] *Full details on the Controlled Scientific Study carried out on Azilect appear in Appendix 4, under 'More information on MAO-B Inhibitors'.*

From the information printed in Appendix 4, I would personally assume that if taking Eldepryl could possibly slow down the progression of Pd, then Eldepryl must have been one of the reasons why my pd started to improve.

Within two weeks of starting to take Eldepryl, I already began to slowly feel better. I was still working at that time, although I was busy handing my job over to my successor. The only aspect of my life that had changed, at that point, was the introduction of the Eldepryl. So, it can safely be assumed that the Eldepryl, on its own, did have some sort of a beneficial effect. **MAO-B inhibitors do not mask symptoms,** as I believe do other forms of Pd medication.

At the time, when the neurologist prescribed the Eldepryl, he said that the manufacturers *claimed* that it could possibly *halt the progression of Pd,* and if I were lucky, I would be able to maintain my present quality of life and not deteriorate any further. It is possible and probable that this has actually happened, and that these tablets have successfully halted the progression of my Pd, together with the Exercise.

Late in 1999, my neurologist decided to put me onto Sinamet, in addition to the Eldepryl, because he felt that my condition was deteriorating. The dosage started with half a tablet twice a day, and worked up to three tablets a day, over a period of approximately one month. Contrary to what he felt about my condition, I felt that it was progressively getting better, but he wanted me to increase my medication. This was quite a blow to me. I thought I was feeling much better, when I went to see him. No! I knew I was feeling much better. I was so upset about this development. It only goes to show the effect of a doctor's diagnosis on the psychological state of a patient. I knew, without any doubt, that I was getting a lot better, because of the reduction in the number and level of most of my symptoms. And then, out of the blue, my doctor told me that my condition was getting worse. I don't think for one moment that he was telling me lies; he is a very professional doctor. I think he must have seen some degeneration in one or more aspects of my Pd that I was either not aware of, or had overlooked.

After taking Sinamet for three months I did not feel any benefit whatsoever. My movement problems had already been solved and the tremor had already disappeared. Sinamet does not mask all of the symptoms of Pd but, those symptoms, which I think it does mask, I was already able to overcome, by using my conscious brain. That being the case, I decided to stop taking it. I do not like the idea of taking any drugs, especially if they do not appear to have any beneficial effect. I have since been told that this is a clear indication that I do not have Pd.

As far as I am aware, all drugs containing levodopa, can and do cause dyskinesia, if too much is taken, and the on/off condition, which gets worse as more is taken, until the time comes when the medication does not work at all.

Twelve months later, on my next and final visit to my neurologist, I told him what I had done and the reasons why I had done it. He did not pass any comment, but I am sure that he did not approve of my action. I had already told him, when he had previously prescribed the Sinamet, that I was not happy about taking that particular type of drug. I was, and still am, under the impression that Levodopa drugs have some sort of a window period, during which, the patient enjoys a very good quality of life but, during that window period, the dosage has to regularly be increased, in order to remain effective, but the side effects tend to increase as well. At the end of that window period, I believe that the body has built up a resistance to the drug, which then ceases to have any positive effect. The side effects by then can be very unpleasant indeed.

More than one neurologist has stated, at various Information Days, which I have attended, that Levodopa medication should be a **last resort medication**, when all other Pd medication has failed. However, I have known many sufferers, who had been prescribed Levodopa medication, right from the very beginning. Is this because some doctors are not kept up-to-date with the latest thinking? Or is it because the Sinamet works so well that the doctors feel that the patient will get the best immediate benefit from it, regardless of the long-term consequences? As a Pd patient I personally think that early prescription of Levodopa medication is irresponsible. That is just my opinion.

I did not want to get into that situation, unless there was no other option. I may be entirely wrong about the Levodopa type drugs but, as a layman, it is very difficult to get a clear understanding of exactly what various drugs do, and what their side effects really are, unless we take note of our own, and other's experiences.

My quality of life has not been bad at all, since six years after the initial diagnosis. I think that I would be foolish to take more medication, under these circumstances, even though the neurologist stated that my condition was deteriorating, and that I should start taking the Sinamet. His diagnosis, and my feelings about my condition, at that time, did not match one another at all. As I have said, it *is* possible that he picked up something, of which I was unaware, or more likely, he felt that after nine years, I would need to take one of the levodopa medications, in order to improve my quality of life. I don't know! All I do know is that, at that time, my quality of life was better than it had been, since long before the time I was diagnosed.

As a result of his decision to put me onto Sinamet, I have chosen not to go back to him or any other neurologist, other than after the book was completed (See The Aftermath, Part 4). You may feel that this was a little high handed on my part, but my reasons seemed quite practical at the time. Long before the end of each year, my medical aid benefits ran out, and I landed up paying for a large portion of my medical expenses, in addition to the medical aid society subscriptions. This is still the same today, and in times of rising inflation and incredible medical cost increases, it is not easy for pensioners to balance their budgets. I am not pleading poverty, but we all have to manage our limited resources in the best way possible, and I would rather take Shirley on a cruise holiday than pay for unnecessary medication, or doctor's consultations.

I would like to stress once again for your own sake, in the strongest terms that:

I do not recommend that patients stop taking their medication, without first discussing it with their doctor.

If you feel that *your* medication has too many side effects, or you are not prepared to put up with any of these side effects, or even feel that you are not deriving any benefit from your medication, I strongly recommend that you **talk to your neurologist**. Rather ask *him* to change the medication, if you are unhappy with it. If he/she is unwilling to change your medication, get a second opinion.

Finding the right Pd Medication for you is sometimes a trial-and-error process, and if you do not give any feedback to your neurologist, it may be assumed that you are happy with it. You have a right to question your medication, but **don't do what I did,** by making rash decisions on my own. At the same time, you should not continue to take medication, with which you are not happy. Rather get a second opinion.

I can understand my neurologist having prescribed the medication as he did. That was the way he was trained to deal with Pd. I should, in all fairness, have gone back and expressed my dissatisfaction and disagreement with his latest diagnosis. I had already started to feel a lot better, at that stage, before he put me onto the additional Sinamet. I felt there was very little it could have done for me, other than give me additional problems. I tend to shy away from confrontational situations, and I find that I get very frustrated when I can't verbalize my feelings in a coherent way, when I am under stress.

Doctors are fallible, and sometimes the communication between doctor and patient leaves a lot to be desired. During my visits to the neurologist, he used to ask me various questions about whether I had this or that symptom. He also conducted various tests. I feel that, if he did not ask the right questions, then he was never going to establish the exact state of my health. Instead of only asking, "Do I have this, or does that happen?" he would have got a better idea of my condition had he asked, **"What changes have you noticed since I last saw you?"** Being schooled in the belief that the overall condition of patients cannot improve, I can understand why he never asked that type of question.

I can only view this problem from my own perspective and experience. We are learning every day about new approaches to the treatment of neurological disorders. Christopher Reeve, before he died in September 2004, was able to move his fingers and toes, after having severed his spinal cord and been made a quadriplegic. This was hard to believe! He firmly believed that he would, one day, walk again and worked hard at this, before he suddenly passed away.

As stated earlier, I had unilaterally stopped taking the Eldepryl, on three occasions, since I was first diagnosed. On the first two occasions, I took myself off because I felt so good, and saw no reason why I needed to take them any longer. This was a mistake, because the symptoms returned very quickly, within six weeks, each time. Then I realized I had to start taking them again, with my tail between my legs.

I took myself off Eldepryl on the third occasion, for a period of ten months, between January and October 2001, because of my seriously high blood pressure, which was possibly caused by the Eldepryl, but I did not know that then. Unfortunately, after that break, most of the symptoms had returned again to, what I felt was, an unacceptable level. By then, I had taken Eldepryl for more than nine years.

Although I was not on levodopa medication, let me express a warning: -

Do not even contemplate suddenly going off levodopa medication, unless you have first consulted your doctor.

As I have stated, the reason I went off the Eldepryl, together with all my other medication, at the beginning of January 2001, was that my dangerously high blood-pressure was thought to have had a chemical cause. The heart specialist had decided that my blood pressure problem could only have been medication related. While the doctors contemplated this problem, I made the decision to stop taking all of my medication, for at least a short while. At that stage, I had no idea which of my medications could have been the problem, and I knew that it could be dangerous without the blood pressure medication, especially the risk of a stroke, but I had to do something. I was prepared to take that risk. I was in a catch-22 situation! Without a change, my blood pressure was so high that a stroke was inevitable. If I came off the medication, how much worse could it get?

Going without the Eldepryl did not worry me too much, as I was prepared to face the effects of not having it for a short while. I thought the worst that could have happened could have been the return of all the symptoms. I still had all the movement symptoms, even though I was able to overcome them. The other symptoms affecting my autonomic nervous system were the ones, which were at risk. However, I knew that I could go back on immediately, should the need have arisen.

I checked my blood pressure every day for over three months. As it turned out, I watched it slowly improve but, still not to an acceptable level. After four months, when I resumed taking the blood pressure pills again, my Pd symptoms had showed no signs, at that stage, of returning to that unacceptable level.

After those four months, without the Eldepryl, at the end of April 2001, I decided that my symptoms appeared to be stable, without the use of Eldepryl. However, during the winter months I got another chest infection and had to stop my aerobic walking, for over three months. This, together with the lack of the Eldepryl, definitely affected the symptoms and they slowly returned again, to an unacceptable level, during September, so I resumed taking the Eldepryl again, on the 1st October 2001. A month later, I made another unilateral decision. I decided to reduce the dosage to one tablet a day, instead of the two prescribed, because the symptoms were not severe and, seeing that I had not needed them for nine months, I felt I could safely reduce the dosage. It was later pointed out to me, by a neurologist, that one Eldepryl a day could do nothing for me, although with one tablet a day, the symptoms did disappear again. Maybe that was due to the placebo effect or even the resumption of the exercise program.

The symptoms, which had deteriorated most, were: depression, lack of coordination, essential tremors, inability to swallow, choking, clumsiness, rigidity, social withdrawal, loss of voice, worse insomnia, constipation and exhaustion.

Some drugs take a long time to become effective, and their effects continue long after ceasing to take them. It is therefore not easy to monitor the effects of any specific medication. Also, it has to be remembered that, other than MAO-B inhibitors, I believe that none of the other Pd medications affect the progression of Pd; they merely mask the symptoms; and if the medication is discontinued, the reappearance of the symptoms does not mean that the Pd has got any worse.

More and more stroke victims are now able to regain the use of their limbs, made useless by the stroke. Some people are surviving more than thirty years, after being diagnosed with Pd, mainly by staying active and doing regular exercise.

I still see articles in the media, in which it is claimed that there are still no medications on the market that are capable of reversing Pd symptoms. If you read the articles quoted in Appendix 4, you will see that this is not true. So, why are these articles still being printed? Are the manufacturers of non-MAO-B inhibitors trying to pull the wool over our eyes, or is it the media that is out of date?

The articles in Appendix 4 say it all!

Chapter 5
Attitude Adjustment

Attitude plays an enormously important role in maintaining overall health, especially when we have a chronic illness. I understand that not feeling well, is reason enough to be negative, but it is exactly under these circumstances that we must endeavor to maintain a *positive attitude.* Over the years, I have addressed many people, at support group meetings. One observation has become very obvious to me:

My experience has been that: we PwPs have been conditioned to accept that, until a new drug arrives, there is *NO HOPE* of any improvement in our condition. We *must* expect our condition to gradually deteriorate, until we become totally immobile.

I refuse to accept this prognosis.

Now that we know that a certain type of Exercise and MAO-B inhibitors can both help to slow down or even reverse the progression of Pd, therefore, **there is no reason any more to tell people that there is still no hope!** I am not in the position to say that nobody has been told about these new developments, but are patients now being told about what they can do to slow down or reverse the progression of Pd? I may be quite wrong in thinking that this news has not filtered down to the neurologists, but I have not heard anything about it, at any of the information days I have attended. **It is not being treated as the great news it really is.**

It would be better if patients were told that: by taking an MAO-B inhibitor and having a commitment to regular exercise, adopting a positive attitude and managing our stress levels, there is a good chance of at least maintaining our present condition, without it getting any worse. So,

Why *is it really necessary in 2010 to tell us there is NO HOPE?*

NEGATIVE thinking generates negativity all around. This negativity spreads to others, and becomes a self-fulfilling prophecy. POSITIVE thoughts tend to generate positive actions. They also generate enthusiasm among other people, with whom we come into contact.

I have never met a successful person who constantly sends out negative vibes.

We all have the occasional negative thought. It is only natural, but we all have to guard against becoming negative in our outlook on life

Adopting a negative attitude towards Pd is the worst possible approach to take. You cannot maintain or improve your quality of life if you believe that it is not possible.

Depression is part of Pd. I believe it to be the worst symptom of this disease, because it takes away our will to fight. It also does something else, equally as damaging, by making the lives of our caregivers very unpleasant. It is one thing for the caregivers to tend to our needs, but it is another, to have to put up with criticism and irritability, from the very people they are trying to help. Not only does depression make us irritable and uncooperative, it gives our caregivers the feeling that what they are doing is futile.

Imagine what difference it would make to the lives of those wonderful caregivers, if we were to proffer a smile or a kindly word, even though we are feeling miserable, instead of complaining. There is no doubt that not only does a cheerful attitude make an enormous difference to the lives of those around us, it also makes a difference to *our* own lives.

I have personally found that a cheerful attitude and regular exercise have a very positive effect on clinical depression. I am sure that your doctor can explain this phenomenon better than I can. Let it suffice to say that it is more beneficial to the body, and the pocket, to adopt this approach to depression, rather than taking pills.

In Chapter 1, Part 1 of the book, I said that, 'I was enjoying the sympathy received from family and friends'. Receiving sympathy is all well and good, and has its place in the healing process, but it is a negative motivation, which causes us to look inwards, and feel sorry for ourselves. **It is so easy to drown in a sea of self-pity.**

Looking back now, I was very lucky to have shaken off this mood of 'Feeling sorry for myself', and I strongly advise all other PwPs, who have yielded to this temptation, to do the same. Not only is it bad for our health, it makes the lives of our caregivers unbearable. I replaced this inward-looking attitude, with a '**What can *I* do?**' approach.

We may feel that we are becoming rather helpless, but we have to be very far down the track before we actually do become helpless. Helping others, would take our minds off our own problems. It also makes us aware of their suffering, which might be far worse than our own. It opens up our minds, and allows new thoughts in.

It is nobody's fault that we suffer from this disorder. There is nobody to blame for our situation. Feeling sorry for ourselves cannot possibly do anything positive for us. It can only make other people want to give us **a wide berth**.

In order to start on a daily program of exercise, we first have to adopt **a positive attitude,** otherwise we would never be able to expect a successful outcome. You will find that **attitude is a habit** and, like most habits, it is difficult to change. But, oh! What a difference it makes when we do. Do you ever get a good feeling, when seeing a disabled person with a radiant smile, or do you get a guilty feeling?

Think of my two heroes; Helen Keller and Douglas Bader, whose attitude made all the difference to their chances of success. When Helen Keller suddenly realized that her mentor had all along been trying to help her, she changed her whole attitude, and started to cooperate with her, instead of selfishly doing the things she wanted to do.

Likewise, when Douglas Bader realized that the only way he could ever fly again, was first to prove that he was as good as anybody else, and to do that, he had to be able to walk unaided, even though that seemed like a total impossibility. The key to their success was a:

POSITIVE ATTITUDE!

'I firmly believe that, other than taking the prescribed medication, you the patient, are the only person in a position to genuinely improve your own quality of life. In order to do this, you must BELIEVE that you *can* do it'.

Chapter 6
Mental Stimulation

Socially, after diagnosis, I became very reluctant to mix with other people, and limited my excursions to close relatives, who knew about my clumsiness and other problems, and understood that I sometimes needed to lie down and sleep. They were not offended by my apparent disinterest in what was going on around me, or even in their conversation.

Those first six years are now, fortunately, quite a blur in my memory, because I did not do very much worth remembering, other than my exercise. I did attend the quarterly company board meetings, none of which stand out in my memory, and I did pop in to see some of the staff, on odd occasions. Shirley and I continued to travel quite extensively, as we had done all our working lives, although, after retiring, it was purely for pleasure. This was of great benefit to me, because it kept my mind alert. Other than the odd game of cards and my computer programming; reading and traveling were the only stimuli my mind received during those six years.

Since 1978, I have been playing cards with a group of fellow Rotarians, in Springs, and although it is over fifty kilometers away, I do still go there and keep the friendships alive.

Many times during this story, I have mentioned that I wrote a suite of programs to run my business. Back in the seventies, I also undertook to write an additional suite of programs, capable of running *any* other type of printing business and this suite also had to be re-written, in preparation for the new millennium. The reason I did this was because all of my customers were printers, and I was certain in my mind that if they became more successful, they would generate more business for my company as well.

Several of my customers persuaded me to do this at a time, when I was feeling a lot better than I had in 1992. The prospect of doing a re-write was quite exciting to me, and being the eternal optimist, I believed that it would not take me longer than six months, so I glibly said yes to their request. I was quite excited about this and found it very stimulating. Eighteen months later, I had still not finished those programs, for reasons that are not important to this story. What is interesting is that I had reverted to the habit of working up to twenty hours a day, in order to get the project finished, before the 31st December 1999. To cut a long story short, I delivered the completed programs in February 2000, and somehow still managed to keep the customers happy.

Having worked such long hours again, under a great deal of pressure, should logically have brought on the symptoms of Pd again. But it didn't. Not only did it *not* surface again, it actually continued to get better. *WHY?* The answer is not easy, and is, at this stage, pure conjecture. The only difference that I am able to establish, between the previous work situation and the new millennium situation, was that I experienced no negative stress. There were no unpleasant phone calls, even when I was overdue. There were no financial or staff problems and definitely no management problems. The key seems to be *the absence of negative stress.*

Programming taught me another positive lesson, which is probably more important than we may think!

I had to use my BRAIN and, in so doing, my brain became a lot more STIMULATED.

Simply stated, a program is a list of instructions, for the computer to carry out, when it is loaded and running. Fortunately, writing computer programs is not the only way to stimulate the brain. There are many more pleasant pastimes, which are very stimulating: -

I.   **Playing Bridge**, or any other card game, involving memory, strategy and intense concentration.
II. **Playing Chess or Scrabble**, or any other board game requiring a lot of concentration.
III. **Playing tennis, bowls or golf**, which require strategy, and provide good healthy exercise, and coordination.
IV. **Reading** helps the brain to create mental images
V.   **Computer games**, which keep the brain and hands active, and exercise our hand/eye coordination.
VI. **Painting and sculpting,** which stimulate the brain, forcing it to analyze everything that is being depicted.
VII. **Handicrafts**, such as woodwork, knitting, sewing etc., for keeping the brain and the limbs active.
VIII. **Play reading,** which is stimulating, and you will be mixing with other people..
IX. **Surfing the Internet,** requiring intelligent interaction.
X.   **Cryptic Crossword and Su Doku puzzles**, which I think are the best ways to stimulate the mind.

XI. **Writing stories**, which compel the brain to create mental images, and turn them into words.

XII. **Voluntary work**. Helping others, takes our minds off our own problems and enriches our lives.

Before I got married in 1960, I became involved in the Kimberley Amateur Dramatic Society (Reps), where I learnt a little about acting, but more importantly, I learnt the importance of theatre in the life of a community. Soon after we married, I was also invited to join Round Table. I soon got involved in putting on stage shows for Round Table, to raise funds for various charities. The most popular shows were 'Melodramas'. These shows included a fair amount of singing, in which the audience participated, giving them a great deal of pleasure. Since then, I have sung on very many occasions, mainly to senior citizens in their clubs and retirement villages, in and around Kimberley, Springs and Johannesburg. This is something I continued to do, for over thirty years, and although I battled a bit in recent years with my words, the old dears still loved it, and didn't mind too much, when I fluffed the words up. They were always happy to see a new face, and to be entertained. The songs I sang were mostly from the period, 1930 to 1970, and were well-known to all of us. In recent years, I have started to get stuck, while singing. It was not because I did not remember the words; I simply got a mental block. Sometimes I could not even think of the starting line of my song, which always left me standing there looking and feeling like an absolute idiot. This happened more and more often, and did not do my tremors or self-confidence any good, at all. Consequently, I gave up the singing in 1999, hoping that I would get over the problem sometime in the future. I have now started singing again, at our retirement village functions, with a reasonable amount of success.

I have a very uncomfortable memory, relating to singing in public. This was at the wedding of the daughter of one of my senior staff members. When the time came to sing John Denver's beautiful ballad, "Perhaps Love", to the young couple. My hands and legs started to shake uncontrollably, and my mouth went completely dry. I soldiered on through that beautiful ballad, until the bride and groom could not contain themselves any longer. They burst into laughter, in front of everybody. They were as unaware as I was of what was happening to me. To them, it was very funny, watching me shaking from head to toe, as I battled to finish, what should have been, a beautiful moment in their young lives. I was devastated! After thirty odd years of entertaining people, I had been reduced to performing a comedy act, in a church, of all places.

Now, in 2010, I am still getting a mental block of some of the words, but I get by. As I have said, in order to capture a little of my singing ability, I have decided to make a CD for my family, because I know so little about my own parents that, to be able to hear one of them sing, or read a story would be very heart-warming to me, in my twilight years. Neither Shirley nor I have ever been able to recall anything about our parents, before we were born. We only have our memories. As young people, we didn't think of that sort of thing. We don't know where they were born, where they went to school, where they worked, or even what they did for pleasure. I feel sure that our children and grandchildren would love to have an audible record of their Pops, in addition to the paintings, photos and old cards etc. I did once set out to write my memoirs, but somehow, never got around to finishing them.

Even if you don't sing or play a musical instrument, why not take up as many activities as you possibly can? These activities should stimulate your mind and get you back into the mainstream of life. Your brain is the part of your body, which is not functioning properly. Brain stimulation makes a great deal of sense and, even if these activities don't have any visible positive effects:

WHAT HAVE YOU GOT TO LOSE?

Chapter 7

The Final Piece Of The Puzzle

Everything mentioned so far, in this process of my 'apparent recovery', has really been common sense. It applies to everybody, not only people with movement disorders. However, there is one change that I made to the way I control most of my movements, which has, I believe, overcame most of the more debilitating effects of my symptoms. This could not have been achieved without having done everything else in Part 2, but I think that this final piece of the puzzle is the **key to my good fortune.**

When I attended Dr Weinberg's seminar – mentioned in Part 1, chapter 2, - I spoke to him afterwards about the improvement in my condition, and he gave me the following explanation, which I am repeating here verbatim. Unfortunately, it is not in layman's language but, like me, I am sure you will understand the gist of it.

Some thoughts on PNI and Parkinson's disease

"Essentially, Parkinson's disease is a degenerative process, involving cells producing dopamine (pathways extending from midbrain to basal ganglia). This type of Parkinson's is termed paralysis agitans, and is the most common type. Interestingly a type of Parkinson's disease occurred in the 1920's as a result of damage to the same system of cells, caused by epidemic viral encephalitis.

I had always assumed that advanced Parkinson's, similar to a stroke, was irreversible, because of loss of actual brain cells. But in your case it showed that nothing should be regarded as irreversible – the process of enhanced wellness and performance through enhancement of mindset is a very powerful and widely permeating process.

Although I direct most of my energies, in terms of PNI, towards immune enhancement, it has become apparent, through sophisticated research, that positively enhanced mind states can also diminish osteoporosis and promote wound healing.

In your list of life situations, which may give rise to suppressed immune function, there is a common trait – that of loss, which leads on to despair and subsequently purposelessness. If the situation is perceived as being irreversible, this then leads to the development of serious pathology (Abnormal changes in body tissue, caused by disease).

In terms of my treatment approach, I believe that the management of the "end-organ" i.e. the organ with the tumor, or the system that lacks adequate chemistry, should be conducted in parallel with the mind (psycho-social) enhancement. "Coming to terms with one's trauma", requires in fact, re-programming the mind-brain. In other words, insert new software (program) to replace defective inherited software, which, through an interaction with the environment, received negative feedback. It is thus the software, which determines our behavior (actions and responses) within the greater environment, which would need to be re-programmed.

It may be a good idea to visit my website at www.pninet.com for further concepts which may be of some help."

The entire medical profession does not necessarily share these views, which have been expressed here by Dr Weinberg. However, he is prepared to look beyond the accepted norms of his profession, and examine other possible causes for mental and physical illnesses, which have troubled mankind for centuries. He has given us a brief insight here into his understanding of the power of the mind.

In the previous chapters, I have spoken about factors that have slowly brought about a general improvement in my condition. But, by the middle of 1999, none of the effects of the symptoms had improved to the level they are at now. At that stage, an important event took place in my life.

I had become accustomed to my 'essential' hand tremor (this tremor occurs, when using limbs on the affected side of the body). This had become part of my life. You can imagine my surprise, when, quite by accident, I found that, if I concentrated on holding my glass firmly in my right hand, I was able to drink out of it *without* the tremor.

Repeatedly, I found that if I held the glass normally, my hand tremor was omnipresent, but if I concentrated on holding the glass very firmly, the tremor disappeared.

Thinking about this at that time; the only possible explanation, that I could come up with, was that I was using my **conscious** brain, when I picked the glass up with a firm grip, because I had to concentrate on what I was doing. I assumed that I was therefore **using a different part of my brain, to control an action, which was normally controlled by my subconscious brain.** All tasks, which are normally done without having to think about them, are controlled by the subconscious brain. The moment we try to do any of these tasks differently, then our **conscious brain** takes over. I call this 'Conscious Control' - John Argue calls this, 'doing things mindfully', see Appendix 3.

Many people find it hard to understand what I mean by doing something **consciously**. They feel that everything we do is done consciously. They are right, but not in the sense of the 'control' of every single movement we make. During most activities, like walking, eating, swallowing, writing and many other repetitive actions, the movements are controlled by our **subconscious** brain. Actions we repeat over and over again, get stored up in our subconscious brain, so that we can concentrate on more important things, while we are carrying out those actions. For instance, when we are walking, we don't think about **how** to walk, we only have to think about **where we are going, and about obstacles in our path.**

Pd affects the subconscious brain's ability to carry out its function properly, because messages do not get to the limbs on time, or even at all.

What we have to do, is **take over the control of all of these functions, by consciously controlling each individual movement.** I don't think that I achieve this completely with everything, but, with eating and drinking I have to concentrate on everything I do, including the swallowing.

This all sounds very complicated and It is; but we have done it all before, when we were much younger. After carrying this out for a month or two, we will find that our necessary level of concentration reduces to a point which, although we still have to think about it, we are able to think of something else at the same time.

The same goes for bringing a glass of water up to the mouth. and getting the water safely into it. If only we had a little switch we could flick, to change from subconscious to conscious. As my grandchildren say, that would be 'cool'.

In order to change over to the conscious brain, I have found it easier to do if I carry out the action slightly differently. By doing this, I automatically change control back from the subconscious to the conscious brain. The same thing happens, when I try to take control of my walking. If I lose concentration, my brain immediately reverts back to the subconscious. I know when this happens, because the bad walking gait returns immediately, and I **can feel the effect of this change**. Practice; practice; practice. That is what is needed, in order to get used to walking, without the bad gait.

More than a year after I discovered how to hold the glass consciously, without spilling anything, I was entertaining another PwP to lunch at my home, when I noticed that he also had a hand tremor, when he lifted his wineglass to his mouth. I asked him to hold the stem very firmly and have another sip, which he did. To his surprise, his hand did not shake either.

I later carried out this experiment with somebody else, but she found it too difficult to hold the glass firmly. As an alternative, I told her to hold the glass differently, such as from behind, instead of from the side. This created the condition, where her conscious brain had to control the action. She also had no tremor, when she drank in this way.

This simple little discovery was the beginning of a process that has changed my life. It was the final piece of the puzzle.

Then, I set about trying to find a way of using my conscious brain to help me overcome other dinner table problems. I soon found that if I held my fork, pointing forty-five degrees towards me, and with a firm grip, I was able to achieve the same result. I found, with a spoon, the harder I held it, the more I shook, when tipping the spoon into my mouth. Why? I don't know. I now hold it very loosely, balancing the weight of the spoon and contents on the end joint of my index finger and loosely using my thumb to hold the end of the handle down to keep it level. The weight of the spoon and contents, are obviously on the opposite end to the thumb.

When I used my conscious brain to control my movements, I noticed that they were performed much more slowly than normal, but they were all much more controlled. Once again, this must have been because I was controlling my actions in a different way to normal. I found that:

In order to be able to control my movements differently to the usual way, I had to use my conscious brain to perform such tasks.

The subconscious brain has been programmed to control many of our repetitive daily activities, but this is the part of the brain that has difficulty in communicating with the body.

People with Pd, like me, who have problems with walking or writing, have to go back to square one and, **consciously learn to control every one of these repetitive actions, and keep on doing so for the rest of their lives.** This is because the Pd can affect every single subconscious movement we make.

We don't all have a writing problem, or a bad walking gait, or struggle to put food and drink into our mouth. If we do have a problem, with any action or movement, which we don't normally have to think about, we can no longer rely on our subconscious brain to control that function.

All actions, such as writing, walking, talking, eating, speaking, riding a bicycle, swimming, riding a horse etc., are controlled by the subconscious brain, after we have learned how to do them. There are other things, like swallowing and breathing etc, which are also controlled by the subconscious brain, but not in the same area as the 'learned' skills. However, we can, and often do, interfere with these functions as well. To illustrate this, I refer to the breathing function. We don't ever have to think about how to breathe, or even when to breathe. However, we can intervene at any time in the breathing process. We can stop breathing, for a while anyway. We can breathe faster, and we can breathe slower. We can even breathe deeper. When we do any of these things, the subconscious brain takes over immediately, if we run short of oxygen. If we have too much, we can actually pass out, but when we do, the breathing returns to normal.

We normally swallow, without knowing. It is automatic, like blinking. These functions can also be affected by Pd. We can swallow consciously, when we are aware that we have a lot of saliva in our mouth. We can blink consciously, when the eyes feel dry. However, this is not practical, and therefore needs medication. When we swallow, the trachea (windpipe) is normally closed, but with Pd, it sometimes happens that the trachea is still open, when we are swallowing food or liquid, and we choke. This can be consciously avoided, but it is very difficult to concentrate on every mouthful we swallow. What I find happens is, when I am eating and am in conversation with someone, I swallow my food, while I am talking, and that creates a lot of problems. I have to concentrate on doing one or the other, but never try to do both at the same time. It is better to not get involved in conversation, while eating. I am only human, and find it very difficult not to take part in general conversation, at the dinner table, especially when we have company. I then have to concentrate very hard on seeing that I don't swallow something while I am talking. I can consciously close my windpipe, before swallowing.

Another problem I had already solved, back in 1968, was my bad handwriting. My writing had become so small and illegible, that I had been forced to start printing everything out, in what we call block letters. In other words, I had learned to write differently. I found out then, before I knew I had Pd, that if I wrote in block letters, I had no problem doing it properly. I did not know that I was using a different part of my brain, to do this. All I did know was:

My hand did not refuse to work properly, when I wrote in block letters, although it did, when I wrote normally.

When we write, we do not normally have to think about *how* to write, we only have to think about *what* to write. The '*how*' is controlled by the subconscious brain and the '*what*' is controlled by the conscious brain.

After Shirley and I had started walking on our own, away from RWFL, in 1998, I started to question why I was not able to walk like everybody else. Up till then, I had been concentrating on walking faster, and not on walking better.

At that point, I had been walking a lot faster than Shirley and, consequently, we weren't walking together. This was at a time, when it ceased to be safe to walk alone on our suburban streets. There is nothing new about crime, especially petty crime, which is often directed at people, while exercising in and around the areas where they live. This happens all over the world, but here in South Africa at the present time, it is possibly a bit more prevalent, and violent.

A sudden spate of robberies in our area, made Shirley feel very insecure. We agreed to continue walking, but we wanted to walk together. She really wasn't happy about holding me back, knowing how important it was to me, but I was equally adamant that she needed the exercise as much as I did. So, we decided to walk together for the first four kilometers, at her pace, after which, I was free to do the last four kilometers, at whatever pace I chose.

What prompted me suddenly to question the awkward way in which I walked?

At that point, I had already known for more than seven years that I suffered from Pd, which after all, was the cause of this awkwardness. So, why start questioning it **then?** The reason was that I then had *time to think* about the problem, whilst walking, at Shirley's slower pace.

I reasoned that, if I had managed to overcome other symptoms, by doing things differently, why couldn't I walk in a different way? I very soon realized that there is only one way to walk properly, so I could not do it differently. The most compelling reason, for me to learn how to walk properly, was because of the awkward way, in which I had been walking, had caused the recent injury to my back. This new injury necessitated the last back operation and also the knee problems. It needed to be addressed as soon as possible. Therefore, I had to try and walk properly again by:

Concentrating on each individual movement.

First, I had to work out what I was, or wasn't doing properly, which was not as easy as it may sound. In fact, I was so busy concentrating on my walking, I was unable to even keep up with Shirley. On reflection, I don't know what I had expected. I literally had to *re-learn* how to walk.

You may well ask, "If I had been walking so well, time-wise, *why did I need to change?* " Other than the injuries, it was a challenge. *I wanted to change,* and if I succeeded, it would help me to overcome the injury problems.

I eventually established that there were three fundamental flaws in the way I walked, which all related to my legs.

1. My left foot had no spring in it, when I walked, because I was not pushing up and forward on the ball of the left foot, when transferring to the right foot, before it came down onto the ground. It also meant I had to keep my right leg bent, in order to avoid hitting the ground as the right foot came past the left foot.
2. My right knee was still being held bent, when the foot touched the ground, instead of being held straight.
3. I was taking unduly short steps.

Problem number one puzzled me for quite a while, because I was able to stand on my toes with ease, so, why did I not have that spring in my left foot, when I walked? For the record, my left calf was considerably smaller than the right, probably because of the pinched nerve on my left side, when I had the original back injury, and this had affected my walking.

While walking, I am able to correct some of the movements, by concentrating on what I am doing, and the rest of the action is still controlled by the subconscious brain. When lifting food or drink to my mouth, I control the whole action, 'consciously'. I am no longer able to simply tell myself to walk, I now initially have to think of activating each movement, one at a time. In order to walk we must first move our weight onto one leg and then lift the other leg off the ground, move it forward, keeping the knee bent, then straightening the knee, when the foot is ready to touch the ground. Just before that point; push up and forward on the ball of the back foot; Then plant the heel of the front foot firmly onto the ground. Then transfer the weight off the back foot and lift it off the ground, bend the knee slightly, and bring the leg forward past the front leg; then straighten the front knee, while pushing up and forward on the ball of the back foot; then planting the heel of the front foot firmly onto the ground.

In practice, I did not have to think about every individual step motion, but only certain parts of the motion, such as pressing up on the ball of my left foot, as the right foot moved past the left foot. I also have to:

- concentrate on keeping the weight of my body on the middle of each foot, as it touches the ground.
- constantly rectify my posture, as I am walking, when I tend to lean forward.
- Swing my arms properly.
- Straighten the front knee, before it touches the ground.

I carry a one-kilogram weight, in each hand, while walking, during my exercise sessions. This helps me to swing my arms properly, without having to concentrate too hard on that function. I also think about each leg, as it passes the other leg, to see that I straighten the knee before the foot touches the ground. These are the actions, which don't occur naturally, while I am walking. I don't know how the brain works, but in my case, the part of the brain that normally controls each of these faulty movements, seems to be damaged in some way.

So, after I realized what I was not doing properly, I was able to consciously push up and forward on my left foot, while transferring my weight to the right foot.

This immediately raised a question in my mind.

Why was the message able to get to the muscle, while I was consciously thinking about it, and not while I walked naturally?

I don't have the answer to this question, other than to say that, if I am using a different part of my brain to walk consciously, then maybe the nerve pathways from that part of the brain are not affected by the Pd.

There has been one important piece of information, which came to me from Mrs. Carole Charlewood, a well-known South African TV personality, who also suffers from Pd. This information gives an important clue to a possible reason why I have recovered so well, since the time of my original diagnosis

Scientists have now proved that the brain also produces dopamine in areas, other than the substantia nigra.

The relevance of this piece of information will become apparent at a later stage. I am not in possession of any medical journal references for this information.

This may not mean too much to you, but to me it suggests that by using the conscious brain, I am using a part of the brain that does not have a shortage of dopamine. Therefore the messages are getting through to the legs and arms perfectly normally, when using my conscious brain.

You will also read, further on in part 4, that others have been able to replicate this phenomenon. Nobody that I have spoken to, up till now, has had any problem using the conscious brain to perform tasks, with either the legs or the arms. More about this later!

Having solved problem number one, the next problem solved itself, when I consciously walked, while supporting my weight on the back foot until the front foot touched the ground. I found that I then had time to straighten my right knee, before the heel actually touched the ground. If I didn't carry my body-weight by lifting upwards on the ball of my left foot, the right foot scraped the ground, unless I kept the right knee bent. So, this problem disappeared when I learned to walk with a spring in my step.

The next idiosyncrasy, which occurred to me, was that I was quite capable of taking a substantial step forward, if I concentrated on doing so, but seemed unable to do it while walking subconsciously. So, what was stopping me from taking longer steps? The answer seemed to be that the awkwardness of my walk made it difficult and clumsy and, because I was prematurely coming down on my right foot, with the knee still bent, I could not lengthen my stride. So, this problem also disappeared when I started walking with a spring in my step.

I have read about this problem, in Pd literature, where it was put down to the fact that, because of lack of use, our muscles are constantly becoming more and more rigid and our tendons shorten, thus reducing the movement of the limbs. Because we develop this 'shuffle', we are unable to walk normally, with the result that we walk less, and the muscles and tendons in our legs shorten and atrophy.

Since I have re-taught myself to walk properly, my stride has lengthened and my leg muscles have developed and become far more flexible.

Not having had any medical training, I have made the assumption that I use a different part of my brain, when I consciously move my legs, to that which I use, when I am walking naturally (Subconsciously). If this is correct, then why doesn't the brain get confused? The mere fact that I make the decision to walk has always been enough to set the brain in motion, in the past, but now I assume that I am overriding that function and am using another part of the brain, to control my leg and arm movements.

When doing my walk in the mornings, I am totally focused on the walking, but with the best will in the world, I often get distracted by outside stimuli, such as other people, and other living creatures. I am a keen birder, and can't resist the temptation to look, when I see movement around me or hear birds call. When this happens, I am made aware of the fact that I am not concentrating, because I immediately feel the awkwardness of my steps and am reminded to start concentrating again on the walking. I find that I am able to talk to someone else, about mundane matters, without losing my concentration, and I don't even lose it if I recognize the birds. This means that I am now able to do multi-tasking, in matters that don't require too much concentration. I don't know that anybody can fully concentrate on two things at the same time;

they can normally concentrate on one task, while doing another subconsciously. In my case, I am consciously thinking of the walking, while subconsciously listening to something else.

The problem comes, when I have to think about something, which has been said, or when I try to conjure up a witty retort. The other more regular distraction is, seeing or hearing an unfamiliar bird, and then wracking my brain, to try to fathom out what it could be. This underlines the fact that I cannot expect to be able to concentrate properly on two different things, simultaneously. It must be quite amusing to walk behind me and observe my erratic passage along a seemingly straight road.

So, I constantly get two different results from the two different methods of walking, and the only way this can happen, in my opinion, is that:

My walking *is* currently controlled by two different parts of my brain.

One part has a problem communicating with my legs and arms, and the other has no problems in this regard.

After having worked all this out for myself, I then spent several months trying to walk, *'heel and toe',* without having to think about it. I have found this to be almost impossible. As I have already said, as soon as I stop thinking about some of my movements, I immediately revert to my old way of walking. And yet, I am now able to eat and drink, without spilling anything, and without knowingly having to think about those actions any more. No, it is not true that I don't spill anything anymore. It is more true to say that, if I am so engrossed in conversation, I still have accidents, and still often choke.

This must mean that I am still consciously controlling the action of feeding myself, while subconsciously listening to the conversation, but the level of concentration is not very high. But when the accidents happen, the control must be flipping over to concentrating on the conversation, while letting the subconscious control the feeding.

As it turned out, there was far more to the foot problems than just walking heel and toe. What I found was that I was supinating, without knowing it. Up until then, I did not even know what the word meant, until the problem was brought to my attention by a podiatrist. He had been asked to find out what was causing the pain in the outside of my knees, while I was walking. He pointed out the wear on the underside of my shoes. It was plain for anybody to see that I was wearing my shoes out very noticeably, on the outside of my right shoe, with no sign of wear on the inside.

When I later succeeded in consciously controlling all the actions of my feet, including walking, with my weight on the centre of my feet, my *balance* problems also seemed to improve. When I failed to pay attention to the positioning of my weight on my feet, by consciously keeping it on the center of the foot, I became prone to *losing control of my balance*, and getting a pain on the outside of my knees.

I think that one of the causes, of my loss of balance, was that my body weight was not always directly over my feet, while walking. When this happened and I was standing on the outside of the foot, the next step was performed, while I was slightly off balance. I have always been led to believe that the loss of balance is due to the Pd. In a way I suppose it is, but not directly. It is, in my opinion, due to **walking badly and also to lack of muscle tone.** If the bad posture and walking can be overcome, then the balance problem will also be mainly overcome; assuming that my muscles are strong enough to do the work. This is the other part to this balance problem. If our muscle-tone is not good, it will have an effect on our balance, because the muscles can't do what is expected of them.

The other contributory factor to the bad gait was the action of walking, virtually *flat-footed,* particularly on the left side. I found that my bodyweight was not being properly supported, when the full weight of my body, was being transferred forwards, onto the right foot. The ball of the left foot was not supporting my weight. The result was that I had no control, when my right foot hit the ground, when I landed hard on that foot, jarring my body and making me aware of the bad gait. This also damaged my spine.

The podiatrist supplied me with an orthotic pad, to put into my right shoe, which was designed to force me to favor the center of the foot, instead of the outside. While walking with this device in my shoe, my walking definitely improved, and the pain I had been getting in the outside part of the right knee, also improved. It was not financially feasible to get an orthotic for every pair of shoes, so I only had it in my walking shoes, and when wearing normal shoes I still supinated.

After all this, I was still aware of favoring the outside of that foot, and it was not long before the pain in my knee returned. I had to consciously walk, while favoring the inside of the foot all the time, not just when doing exercise, if I were to overcome this problem. I still do this, and now my left foot has also developed the same problem, so I have to concentrate on both sides. I had to strengthen the outside calf muscles. Maybe, the Pd was becoming bilateral, which is what my neurologist had picked up. But he did not tell me this.

The problem I had with walking over uneven surfaces disappeared, when I made sure that I was supporting my weight properly on the ball of the rear foot, until the other foot touched the ground. The moment I forget to support my weight on the rear foot, I felt the awkwardness of my walking, and tended to stumble.

There were six other fundamental walking problems:

1. My body was bent forwards, at the hips.
2. My head faced down towards the ground.
3. I was not swinging my right arm.
4. My shoulders were slumped forwards and to the left, so that my head hung slightly to the left-hand side.
5. My right arm was held bent, at a right-angle and tight against my waist.
6. My right hand was held in the shape of a tent and the thumb was held rigidly at right angles to the hand. (Not that this affected the walking)

These problems were fairly easily solved, by consciously correcting each of the faults. However, thinking about all these actions simultaneously to the foot problems, only exacerbated those problems. I am sure that I am not alone in finding difficulty thinking about several things at the same time, in a dynamic situation like walking. To begin with, I found I achieved this, by first getting my posture right, and then concentrating on the arms and feet in rotation. I then checked each movement as it happened, and also the posture. This was quite tiring, and made it very difficult to even think about anything else, while I was walking.

On the lighter side! This *focused* concentration, got me into trouble. One of my erstwhile friendly neighbors tore a strip off me, when I stopped to talk to him one morning. He said I had passed right by him on two previous occasions, with my nose in the air, without even so much as a nod. He was visibly upset and very serious, and gave me a piece of his mind. He did not want to accept my apology and told me to leave him alone. I was dumfounded! I normally greet everybody I pass, while on my walks, this accusation seemed totally misplaced. However, two days later, I stopped and told him about my Pd and what I was doing to overcome it. He found my story difficult to believe, but, he was obviously in a better frame of mind, and accepted my apology. I place a strong value on common courtesy, and made sure that I kept a lookout for anybody I knew; so that this never happened again.

Talking about concentrating on my actions, I must warn anybody who wants to give it a try; that **it is not easy**, and it will take a long time before it will come right. Just remember, that while you are doing all this, your body and brain are getting a great deal of benefit from it, and you will feel that benefit in time to come.

I don't pretend to have studied anything about the brain, or how it works. Everything I say is based on my personal observations and facts I have learned at Information Days, as a PwP, and should be viewed as such.

If we choose to go the route of learning to use the conscious brain, to control faulty movements, we have to get used to using our conscious brain again, as we did as children, learning new tasks. We have to concentrate very hard on our actions and, to begin with, get used to doing them very slowly. This is very tiring, and it requires a lot of adjustment to our thinking. We have to get used to thinking about everything we do, and we have to be patient. When I lose my concentration, my movements become very clumsy and erratic again, thereby prompting my mind to concentrate on what I am doing. That often happens at the dinner table, when I become so engrossed in conversation, I often knock or pull my glass over, or pull the knife or fork off my plate, onto my lap, together with their contents. When walking around the house, thinking of anything but walking, I bump into doorframes, corners of walls, the leg of the bed and/or other furniture. I still trip over carpets indoors and uneven outdoor surfaces. These accidents invariably bring me right back to earth, when I least expect it. However, I am getting more used to concentrating on what I am doing, and treat the odd occasion, when I have an 'accident' as part of life. I don't let these accidents get me down. I try to laugh about them, when I tell my family, and we are all more relaxed about my Pd now.

Since starting to use my conscious brain, to control my movements, my overall condition has improved to the point, where I am more or less free of the debilitating effects of most of my movement symptoms.

I have been amazed at how easy it has been to show patients how to use their conscious brain, to control their walking and bring food and drink to the mouth, without spilling anything. Unfortunately, knowing all this, is only the beginning. Unless the patient is determined to use this knowledge, and concentrate on it all the time, he or she will carry on walking badly, and spilling food.

We have to practice it all the time, not every now and again.

I can now walk, without fear, over uneven surfaces, providing that I concentrate on supporting my weight on my back foot, otherwise the front foot stumbles.

Not until I had succeeded in walking properly, did I think of questioning **why** I could walk properly, when *concentrating* on my movements.

This conscious control of my actions seems to have had some affect on my brain, which is not due to the exercise itself, but to the learned control of that exercise.

This is way beyond my ability to understand, but it is not beyond my ability to recognize. My family and my friends are all very well aware of the change in my condition, even though my condition hasn't been anywhere near as bad as the majority of other sufferers, whom I have got to know since 1997.

Part 3
Thoughts and Actions
Chapter 1
Side Effects Of Medication

What I have been led to understand and have experienced, after many years of health problems is; when we take any medication, we must expect to experience certain side effects. After all, medicines are all toxic. Like many people, I have been taking a cocktail of drugs every day for many years, and have experienced various other health problems - Meniere's Syndrome, asthma, osteoarthritis, back problems – which could have been caused by my medication. My high blood pressure was, I am sure, a side effect of the Eldepryl.

Added to this serious side effect, I have had a larger than usual mammary gland remove from my right side. It was not removed because of its size or appearance, but because it was uncomfortable, to the point of being painful. Discomfort and pain, I believe, are not uncommon to young girls going through puberty, but not being female and certainly not going through puberty, I was advised to have it removed. I was told that this problem was caused by one of my blood pressure tablets. My blood pressure problem was, no doubt, caused by the Eldepryl tablets. (See under Medication in Part 2)

Another side effect, which has occurred over the past seven years, has given me a bit of a scare. My skin became very photosensitive. I cannot sit outdoors, without a hat, and plenty of suntan cream, all over my exposed skin, because my lips and skin come up in peculiar lumps, and my lips break out in sores, which are not fever blisters (Herpes). I am worried that this could turn into something far more serious.

Only one of the side effects had to receive surgical treatment, but that did not make the others any less disturbing. I have gradually experienced a total loss of libido over the past eighteen years, which might be Pd related, or have been due to medication. It was impossible for me to nail this one down, although, at least one of my tablets warned of this possible side effect, in the small print. Fortunately for me, the libido normalized, more or less, five years ago, for a period of three years. Although this was one of the least important benefits, I had gained during this period, it was probably responsible for helping me to regain my self-confidence, and it certainly had helped to put the smile back on my face!

We, as lay-people, stand very little chance of understanding the small print, which accompanies all medication, but that surely is the responsibility of the pharmacist, who should safeguard us from these problems.

I have found it necessary, on two separate occasions, during the past few years, to intervene personally, before actually taking certain conflicting medications, which I would otherwise have taken, with unknown consequences. The pharmacist, and the ENT specialist involved, both apologized for the oversight, and replaced the tablets with more suitable medication. I have not had any medical training, but I have become used to most of the terminology, especially when it comes to Pd. So, it is worthwhile reading the small print, especially if we experience side effects, after taking new medication. The problem is that the side effects do not necessarily show up immediately, and sometimes take months, or even years to manifest themselves. Besides which, who knows when a medical problem is a side effect of medication. We don't carry a medical dictionary around in our heads, and we should never refer to medical books every time we get an ache, or a new type of pain. We are completely in the hands of the medical profession, which is where we should be. At the same time, we should not have to worry whether they are doing their jobs properly, especially when it comes to medication.

Our GP's should take an active interest in all of their patient's medication, including those prescribed by specialists, and act as a clearing-house for the drugs, before we actually take them. However, I think that this is a bit of a pipedream. All the GP's, I have ever had the pleasure of consulting, have been far too busy to undertake this onerous task and, especially in a third world country like ours, we have to accept final responsibility for our own welfare. So, get used to reading the small print and don't feel shy to consult your pharmacist or doctor, if you are not happy about your medication.

The problem appears to be that my GP knows what medication he has prescribed and also knows every time he refers me to a specialist. In turn, each specialist initially asks what medication I am taking. This is where the loophole occurs, in the case of chronic illness. I never think of updating the specialist's records, about my other current health problems and the medication I am taking for those problems. I had Meniere's Syndrome for several years before the Pd was diagnosed and, because of moving residences, I changed my ENT specialists three times over those years, so, records could have become outdated during that period of time.

At present, I take only one pill for blood pressure (previously three). My blood pressure appears to be settling down now, but we are watching it very carefully.

The Meniere's Syndrome stayed stable for over ten years, even without any medication. It raised its ugly head again in 2009, giving me several bouts of giddiness and vomiting.

After I was diagnosed with Pd, I queried the Meniere's diagnosis as well. The specialist, who was handling the case at that time, asked a visiting ENT professor, from the USA, to have a look at it. He also appeared to be uncertain about the diagnosis, but felt that everything pointed in that direction. As I have met many other PwPs with similar hearing and balance problems to mine, I wonder if Pd can affect our hearing.

When I am with other PwPs, I make a habit of asking them what other medical problems they have, but this is a very personal question, and not too many people are prepared to discuss this issue with a layman. My reason for asking this question is that I find it too coincidental that there are a fair number of PwPs around who have three of the same chronic problems that I have. This may not be so coincidental, if we consider that Pd and osteoarthritis are both closely related to ageing and should not be viewed as unusual, but the Meniere's Syndrome is not age related; that is, if it really is Meniere's.

It would be interesting to find out what other medical problems PwPs have in common, which may be more than just coincidence. It could possibly help in the search for a cure for Pd, or some of these other problems. Perhaps this could be a research subject for the future. I have not got a clue as to how one would go about gathering this information, but it is possible in this day and age, and should be investigated.

Chapter 2
Possible Causes Of Pd

I must stress that I am not qualified to talk on this subject either, but, as a sufferer, I have a vested interest in Pd. My experiences, together with all other sufferers, could have a very real influence on the search for a cure for Pd. The thoughts expressed here are purely my own.

There is at least one known cause of Pd, or Pd symptoms, which I have come across, from two totally unrelated sources.

While I was in Port Elizabeth, at a PASA AGM, I had the pleasure of meeting a beautiful young lady from the small town of Potchefstroom, who, together with her twin sister, was diagnosed with Pd at the age of twenty-five. They were caught in aerial crop spraying, in the farming area, where they lived. That was in 1988, and they now face the prospect of going through the rest of their lives, with this debilitating disease. The sister that I met, has a very positive attitude, and has not given in to her quite severe disability. She actively takes part in cycle racing and is keen to get a group of fellow PwPs to do a long-distance ride around the country, to raise funds for Pd research. I did not want to quiz her, but I did wonder whether her doctor or neurologist followed up on the crop-spraying incident, and whether anything was done about it, or anything learned from it.

By strange coincidence, at the same time, I was reading a book entitled "Fields of Air', by James Byrom, which was about the triumphs, tragedies and mysteries of civil aviation, in Southern Africa. I came across this narrative about two unusual accidents, the causes of which had been put down to pilot error. I quote:

"The board found that the accidents were caused by errors of judgment on the part of the pilots, caused solely by the toxic effects of insecticides.

In his report, Dr Gilliland, Chairman of the Board of Enquiry, said that the effects on the central nervous system of the toxins were apprehension, giddiness and emotional lability[8] which would have a serious effect on the pilot's judgment, and could easily result in an accident.

---

[8] Instability.

'The latter effects of insomnia, tremors and difficulty in concentration and poor memory will make the pilot incapable of handling his plane. It is to be noted that these effects may be vague in the earlier stages and become prominent after more of the toxic materials are ingested or inhaled during air spraying,' Dr Gilliland said[9]."

As a layman, it was not too difficult for me to see the similarity of the above symptoms, to some of those of Pd, and the following questions obviously came to mind: -

1. Did those pilots actually have Pd, or did they merely have some of the symptoms of the disease, (Parkinsonism)?
2. Does the young lady from Potchefstroom really have Pd, or do both sisters have Parkinsonism?
3. Has this happened to other pilots anywhere else in the world? If so, were any of them able to be successfully treated, before they also killed themselves? If the answer is yes, can those remedies be used successfully for Pd?
4. Can we contract these same symptoms from food that has recently been sprayed with organic phosphate?
5. How long does it take for crops, sprayed with organic phosphates, to cease being poisonous to human beings?
6. Are facts about organic phosphate poisoning made freely available to the public?
7. I have heard eminent neurologists say, and have also read books, in which it has been stated that, **approximately 25% of all the patients diagnosed with Parkinson's disease have received an incorrect diagnosis,** due to the extreme difficulty in making a correct diagnosis. Do these 25%, of wrongly diagnosed Pd sufferers, fall into the category of people who have ingested or inhaled organic phosphates, or other harmful chemicals?

There are no readily available answers to some of these questions. But answers relating to food, which we eat, are obviously available. In the case of the two young ladies from Potchefstroom, and the two pilots mentioned in James Byrom's book, the correlation of the illness with the crop spraying was not in question. What has been done about it? If nothing, then

---

[9] Pages 286 and 287 in "Fields of Air" by James Byrom.

why has nothing been done about protecting people from this very real danger? Does anything prevent people, who live in the vicinity of crop spraying, being poisoned by these chemicals, as the twins were? I have read many books on Parkinson's disease, and in a few of them, reference is made to the link between crop-spaying chemicals and Pd. Why is this allowed to continue?

My memory and concentration problems could be age related, but the same problems mentioned, in the above extract from Dr Gilliland's report, were probably not about men of my age, but rather about active pilots. Pilots in those days all tended to be younger men, and today that still applies, especially to crop spraying pilots. The reason why I mention this is that these two symptoms may not be specifically Pd related, but may point to the effects of chemical ingestion or inhalation. I do not know if scientists have positive proof, that the memories of PwPs are worse than those of non-Pd people of the same age. The same question has to be asked about their ability to **concentrate.**

Carbon monoxide poisoning also appears to affect the central nervous system. This must be common knowledge.

Chapter 3

General Comments

As the objectives of private enterprise and academia are different, I would expect that the bulk of research, done by the latter is being directed at the cause, rather than the symptoms of Pd. Although, I have no first-hand knowledge on this subject, I feel that there *should* be more interaction between patients and scientists, in addition to the ongoing study and experiments carried out on the brains of deceased patients.

However, I wonder if there is any communication between patients and research scientists? I can imagine it would be difficult for scientists to communicate with non-medical patients. But, if they don't ever talk to patients, then how do they know whether what they are doing is really relevant? This may be a stupid question, but that is how I learn. Doctors and scientists may have all their facts, neatly and accurately stored away in their minds, but does that constitute a total understanding of a subject like Pd? My feeling is that it does not. The human factor may be missing from this equation. The only way to keep the human factor in mind, while doing research, is to keep in contact with the actual patients.

How can one person's memory be compared to that of another? How can my concentration levels be measured against the norm? What is the norm? How can loss of memory, due to age, be compared to loss of memory due to the effects of chemical ingestion? Are the effects of age on the brain, the same as the effects of chemicals?

There are so many questions, which cannot be answered in this book. I also wonder why a benchmark Pd diagnosis has not yet been developed. I am led to believe that the only positive proof of the diagnosis can be obtained from an autopsy. This does not seem to be acceptable in this day and age.

Although medication is absolutely essential at this stage, is too much emphasis not being placed upon it? Are we not too reliant on medication, while not paying enough attention to commonsense issues, such as attitude, diet, exercise and managing stress levels? Are we giving enough thought to the dangers associated with the side effects of medication? Are we doing enough to help patients take an active responsibility for their own health, through appropriate exercise and an informed mental attitude?

The gist of what many patients are told by their neurologist, when they are diagnosed, goes like this:

Accept, and learn to live with this incurable, progressively degenerative neurological disease. Take the recommended medication and live in hope that a cure will be discovered in your lifetime.

This was my experience, and that of many other PwPs I have met. I accept that the doctors and neurologists are technically correct, but from my personal experience, this advice was so de-motivating and soul destroying that **it almost destroyed me.** If patients accept that there is no hope for them, then they will, in all probability, make no effort at all to help themselves. The resulting negative attitude can only be damaging to the patient and family.

Instead of filling patients with visions of *doom* and *gloom*, the medical profession *could* try to help newly diagnosed PwPs *take responsibility* for their own physical and psychological well being, which, together with the *correct medication*, will go a long way towards staving off the ravages of Pd.

I have had Pd symptoms for more than forty-five years (2010), and although I still have most of them, my quality of life is as good as most other people of my age. Whilst trying to assess what my **present symptoms** are, I have taken my age of 75 into consideration. This is the list of my present symptoms, which I regard as being Pd or medication related:

1. Bad muscle co-ordination.
2. Constipation.
3. Choking and swallowing problems.
4. Rigidity and limited movement of limbs.
5. Insomnia.
6. Poor balance, when exercising.
7. Congestion in the chest.
8. Inability to handle stress and conflict.
9. Inability to walk over uneven surfaces, or on carpets, unless I am concentrating hard on what I am doing.
10. Inability to write normally in a cursive script.
11. Inability to find words, and form sentences, especially when tired.

12. Clumsiness.
13. Frequent nighttime urination.
14. Sudden urges to urinate, which are not always real.
15. Fatigue.
16. Poor concentration.
17. Eyes go out of vertical alignment.
18. Hand and leg tremors, on waking up.
19. Profuse perspiration, when performing simple physical tasks.
20. Lack of awareness of temperature, thirst and hunger.
21. Bad walking gait, when not concentrating.
22. Bad memory.
23. Emotional instability. I cry very easily, even while singing songs.
24. Rigidity, after sitting or walking.
25. Inability to multi-task.
26. Loss of voice.
27. Mood swings.
28. Watering eyes.
29. Movements are jerky, when exercising.
30. My toes curl up very tightly (Probably dystonia).
31. Painful leg and foot cramps, mainly at night.
32. Lack of organizational ability.
33. Biting through my bottom lip with my right eyetooth, and through my inner cheek with my back molars.
34. Confusion with which is the right and left side.
35. My calves become flexed, when sitting.

This may sound like a lot of symptoms, but they really do not cause me any serious problems. The only symptoms that give me cause for concern are the severe chest infections, which I seem to get every winter, and the swallowing and choking problems. The last chest infection, and several previous ones, came very close to turning into pneumonia. I have had to take up to five courses of antibiotics, in the past, to bring the infection under control. These chest infections occur because, I believe, my lungs and trachea are not being continually kept clear of phlegm, which is Pd related. I do have to take care that I get enough sleep and don't overdo my activities. In other words, I have to take life a bit easier than I used to.

What's new?

Part 4

The Aftermath

This is the third edition of this book, which has been very well accepted over the past seven years; even though I have not advertised it anywhere. However, the medical profession, generally, has found it very difficult to accept that it has been possible to change the progression of my Parkinson's disease, by taking an MAO-B inhibitor, doing regular energetic exercise and changing my lifestyle.

In the first edition, I made the claim that nobody would ever know that I have Pd, and I decided, before publishing, to put that claim to the test. The neurologist, who had never seen me before, examined me by doing certain checks, but never asked me what my existing symptoms were, or what I had had in the past. He only made certain checks that he considered to be enough to rule out Pd; but he did not test for the cog-wheel effect. I cannot argue with this procedure, as I would think that he should know what he is doing.

After his examination, he made the following statement:

"You exhibit no symptoms of Pd, and it is quite obvious that you never had it in the first place. You had what is known as Parkinsonism, which could have been caused by medication or by another chemical source, possibly crop spraying chemicals".

He asked me what medication I had taken, over the years, and after going through all those I could remember, he singled out one medication, which I took for the Meniere's Syndrome. He said it could possibly have caused the Parkinsonism. He did not elaborate on this, either to tell me whether Parkinsonism is curable, or whether It would have gone away on its own, when I had stopped taking that medication. Most of my symptoms have improved, and some have actually disappeared; but others have continued to worsen.

I tried desperately to remember when I had first taken the suspect capsules for the Meniere's, and the closest I got to the starting date was 1971, a year after I moved from Kimberley to Springs, when the Meniere's Syndrome was first diagnosed. I last took those capsules in the mid 1980s. As at least two of my Pd symptoms started long before 1971, I have no doubt that these capsules had nothing to do with my Pd. My bad writing got to the point that nobody could read my handwriting in 1968, when I had to start printing everything in block letters. The muscle coordination problems had already surfaced, long before that time.

This neurologist seemed quite annoyed that I should have come to waste his time, and he was very abrupt. I was quite dumfounded by his attitude. I did not self-diagnose my condition. I did not prescribe the medication for those past ten years. Did he really think the two previous neurologists did not know what they were doing? Maybe he did not believe that I had actually been diagnosed with Pd in 1992? Why did he get so annoyed? The only conclusion I can come to, is that I present a threat to the medical profession. If all his Pd patients got to a stage, where they no longer need medication, nor to need a neurologist any more, then I can understand his fears.

Should the neurologists not be excited that someone has been able to reverse the progression of Pd? Is it not worth investigating? Why should his reaction have been to get on his high horse?

His diagnosis did not surprise me, because I did not expect him to find any symptoms, other than the 'Cogwheel effect". However, I became quite agitated, when I got back home that day, and had time to think about what had just happened.

I understand, from neurologists, that as many as **25% of all PwPs diagnosed throughout the world, do not actually have Pd**, mainly due to the nature of Pd and other similar related conditions. There is a difficulty in conclusively diagnosing Pd. At present, no definitive diagnosis can be made from X-rays or brain scans, and all diagnosis is based on clinical observation. Many symptoms are shared with other conditions, and none of them can be used as a clear indication of any specific disease. They all get treated as Pd, unless the doctor suspects that it might be something else. I therefore understand this dilemma, but why not point this out to patients, instead of saying, "You definitely have Pd!"

How many people have given up on life, because they thought they had an incurable degenerative neurological disease, when they possibly did not?

I immediately thought, assuming that I might only have Parkinsonism, how many other people, who fall into this 25% category, could possibly have achieved what I have, if they only knew what I know? I don't believe that I have Parkinsonism, but I wondered if anybody else, who does have it, has ever 'got better'?

I realize that I should be very happy, that he thinks I don't have Pd. But **what has changed?** I still have to continue exercising and concentrating on all my movements. I still have to be very careful, when eating and drinking. I still trip, while going up and down stairs and while walking on uneven surfaces, unless I concentrate very hard on what I am doing. I still feel the need for some form of medication, to deal with the insomnia and mood swings. In other words, **my situation has not changed in any way; other than the fact that I am a lot better.**

Shirley and the rest of the family were absolutely incredulous, when I told them what had happened. I also told them that the same neurologist had **taken me off the Eldepryl**; because he said that one tablet a day could not possibly be doing me any good. However, he may have done it because of the blood pressure problem. My family was absolutely astounded. They were as aware as I was that I had already done this on three previous occasions, only to suffer a relapse each time, and they did not want it to happen again.

There was no difference between me and any other PwP. That was until my condition started to improve. The stated motivation for his diagnosis was that;

Because there is no cure for Pd, I could not possibly have had Pd in the first place. Not that I claimed to be cured!

He did not take the time to ask me about everything that has happened to me over the previous ten years. Although he knows a great deal more about this disease than I do, it does not mean that I am not in a position to question his diagnosis.

If I did not have Pd, then the Eldepryl should have caused some serious problems? Surely, a drug, which increases the dopamine levels in the brain, should have caused dyskinesias, in a person who does not have Pd?

There are still some things none of us knows about Pd, and we should not close our minds to anything, regardless of how ill-informed it may appear to be, on the surface. Had he asked me questions about the symptoms I still have, and what I have been doing to overcome many of them, then I would have had more faith in his opinion.

Before printing the book, I gave proof copies of the book to - two office bearers in the Parkinson's Association South Africa (PASA), a leading neurologist at a teaching hospital and a past Director of PASA - for their opinions. None of them came back to me with any negative comments, other than the feeling that "I did not seem too sure about whether I had Pd or not", which, was understandable. I had not said I was not sure I had Pd anywhere in the book, although I had added, at that stage, the details of the incident with the neurologist, and maybe that had raised the doubt as to whether I had Pd. I was still the Chairman (President) of PASA at the time I published the book.

At the next AGM of PASA, after the book was published, I was asked, by the vice chairperson, to not offer myself for re-election, as I had been in the chair for several years. She said that it was not good for an organization to have the same chairman, year after year. I agreed with her and did not offer myself for re-election. This same lady was then elected to the chair. In her first address, after taking over the chair, she did not even thank me for the service I had given the Association, over those past few years, as is normally the custom. In fact her attitude towards me appeared to be quite hostile.

Not long after that AGM, I received a fax from the Director of PASA, asking me to resign. The reason for asking me was that I had used the Association to market my book, which was a load of rubbish. In fact, that same director had asked me, before publication, if PASA could market the book, in order to raise much-needed funds, to which I had agreed. Very strange!

After this, I asked for a meeting with the Chairperson, the Director and the neurologist, to all of whom I had previously given one of the proof copies of my book, before it was published, and all of whom had been asked for their comments. At this meeting, after a lot of discussion, I was told by the neurologist that the problem was that I had a conflict of interests. I was selling the book to members, after meetings, and that conflicted with my position as Vice Chairman. I agreed that it could appear that way, and gave them my resignation the following day. Who did they think I was going to sell the books to, when I gave them the proof copies?

At the next AGM of the Association, the Chairperson got up at the beginning of the meeting and, without any warning, proceeded to read out a statement, condemning me and my book, saying among other things that I: misled people; claimed to be cured; and claimed the endorsement of my book, by the Association. This was also a load of rubbish.

Two of the top neurologists in South Africa were also at that meeting. One of them got up, immediately after this statement was read out by the Chairperson and said that I claimed to be cured, without the use of medication. I questioned her on this point, asking where in my book did I make this claim? She said that, although I did not say this in the book, it was the impression she got after reading it. How can I fight that one? It is interesting to note that none of this appeared on the agenda of that meeting and none of it appeared at the next AGM, in the minutes of the previous meeting. So, I have to conclude that this was a hatchet job, and I was being targeted, but by whom, I am not quite sure.

Who paid the expense of these neurologists to come to that meeting? Why did these proceedings not appear in the agenda or the minutes of that meeting? I am afraid that we all have to draw our own conclusions on this matter.

I have been told that several other neurologists have said, to their patients, that I do not have Pd, when I have not even met them, or even been examined by them. It is possible the doctors have been talking amongst themselves and seem to be very worried about the effect this book is going to have on patients. This might be very innocent on their part. They might well be worried about their patients being led astray by it, but if this is the case, then why the cover-up by PASA?

I don't know how other patients would have handled this situation, but I am no longer able to think on my feet, when things like this happen and I shy away from conflict. I do not have the self-confidence any more to fight this type of attack, and I am sure that others will understand this.

Why am I telling you all this? It is obvious to me, and to many of the people, to whom I talk, that the medical profession has a serious problem with me, and my book. If they feel this way, then why do they not go into the whole matter and be done with it. The answer seems to be that they obviously do not want to.

Needless to say, my dealings with PASA are non-existent any more. I still visit all the support groups, at my own expense, and I still communicate with hundreds of patients throughout the world, on a regular basis. I have not given up on my plan to get the book out to as many people as possible. The costs of going to all those meetings has not been covered by the money received from the sales of the book, so what have I personally gained by doing all this? I am now creating a website to market the book, and hope that this will bring my news to many more people, throughout the world.

The medical profession's attitude is possibly understandable, but not defensible. The only losers, as a result of the actions of those neurologist's and PASA, are *you*, the patients. You don't know what to think about what I have told you in the book. You are left completely in the air.

After I had finished writing the first edition of this book, I asked my family doctor to read and authenticate my story, and write a short foreword, which he so graciously did.

I then set about trying to get some sponsorship, while I looked for a publisher. It took me many phone calls to find out who marketed Eldepryl in South Africa, because it played such an important part in my 'apparent recovery' process, The Pharmaceutical Industry seems to be very secretive, and it took many phone calls to make contact with the person responsible for marketing this product. After nearly six more months, this person put me onto the manufacturers in Scandinavia, with whom I immediately made contact. I thought that they would be overjoyed to hear what part their medication had played in my improved condition, and because of this, I thought they stood to gain a great deal from the book's publication. I remembered what the neurologist had said in the beginning: "The manufacturers claimed that the tablets could possibly halt the progression of Pd". I have still not had a reply from them, after sending them a digital draft of the book, which they requested to see.

I also approached the Run/Walk for Life organization, as they played a major role in my 'apparent recovery'. Here again, I thought that they would be overjoyed at my news, and the part I think they had played in my improved condition. The head of the organization said that they have had many good results with other chronic disorders and were very pleased for me, but could not offer to sponsor the book, because they would be inundated with requests from all over, for sponsorship of various other worthy causes.

Thirdly, I approached my Medical Aid provider, whom I thought would stand to gain a great deal, if only a small percentage of their members with Pd were able to derive some benefits from what I have written in this book. This request also turned out to be very disappointing. They first did their homework, and got a panel of doctors to check into the validity of my claims. They came back to me and expressed certain reservations about one or two aspects of the book, which I was immediately able to change, without altering the story in any way. They were worried that the book might create the impression that I was claiming to have a cure for Pd, although I never intimate that anywhere. Most importantly, they were perturbed about the risk of **falsely raising the hopes of other PwPs.**

I have done my best, throughout the book, to alleviate these fears, by putting appropriate warnings in as many places as possible. Part of this company's marketing drive is to encourage regular physical exercise. They equate regular physical exercise with good health, and give points on a marketing scheme, which can be converted into other material benefits. I felt that my story fitted very well into their approach to avoiding health problems but, regardless of this, they have unfortunately declined to help me with this project, without giving any reasons.

There could be a danger, if patients were deviated from a conservative approach to the management of Pd. I do not argue with this possibility, although **I do not agree with it**.

Another problem I have had is that I have approached three physiotherapists, asking them to write a short article, as an appendix to the book, outlining what they feel about the recommended exercises, and what health benefits patients will derive, if they carry out these exercises. All of them ceased returning my calls, after reading the book. I did not want to embarrass them by physically calling on them for an explanation of this peculiar behavior. Have the doctors, with whom they work, warned them off being involved with something so far-reaching? If they feel that patients would be ill advised to read the book, why not tell me, before I do any damage?

The only actions I am recommending are: to undertake regular exercise and to take the MAO-B Inhibitors, both of which can possibly slow down or even reverse the progress of Pd; adopt a positive attitude; and get rid of all negative stress. In fact, every single adult alive today could take heed of this advice, other than the medication, and put it into practice, without any harmful effects. In addition, I recommend that patients, who have movement problems, **practice using the conscious brain to control those movements**.

Maybe the idea of patients getting better, does not go down too well with the medical profession, although I don't believe that. I could understand the pharmaceutical industry not being happy with what I have said in the book, but overall, the patients would be a lot better off than being without this knowledge.

I have been attempting, for over two years, to motivate a controlled scientific study, on the effects of a combination of - energetic exercise and the use of an MAO-B Inhibitor – as an effective way of treating Pd. Because, applying the benefits of this approach to any specific component of the test, would be impossible. I have to accept that this will never happen. If the Pd world knew, that they could benefit very much from knowing what has happened to me, then there must be some way of going about proving it.

I sincerely believe that we can all learn a lot from what has happened to me. On the one hand, we know about the brain producing GDNF, which repairs damaged brain cells, when we do certain forms of energetic exercise. On the other hand, we know that taking an MAO-B inhibitor can and does also slow down the progression of Pd. The combination of energetic exercise and an MAO-B inhibitor have, in my case, appeared to have brought about a big improvement in my condition. This combination has not cured my Pd, but it has reversed the symptoms enough to give me a very acceptable quality of life.

If every Pd patient took my route of treatment and derived the same benefits as I have, then the search for a cure would become far less imperative.

If enough PwP's are prepared to try this approach to dealing with Pd, and actually get some positive benefit from doing this, then a controlled scientific study would not be necessary. However:

I feel that, unless neurologists advise their patients to do energetic exercise, and also prescribe an MAO-B inhibitor, it has no chance of getting off the ground. This would be such a waste of knowledge and experience.

I appreciate that our most important thrust must be towards finding a cure for Pd, But while we go about trying to reach this elusive goal, we could help millions of sufferers to lead a healthier lifestyle and possibly live a normal life, free of most of the more debilitating symptoms, as I do.

The editor of SPRING Times made a very pertinent observation, during some discussions we have been having by email. He said that it is all well and good knowing that energetic exercise can, and does, help us, if we **can't persuade anybody to do it**. My feelings are that: very few Pd patients will ever do energetic physical exercise **unless their doctor recommends it**, and no doctor is going to recommend it unless it has been properly tested and proven in more double blind scientific studies. A real catch 22 situation!

There are two answers to this objection. Firstly, most newly diagnosed patients *are* **capable** of doing regular energetic exercise! Secondly, it should be recommended that all exercise should start with gentle movement, and *slowly* build-up to maximum levels, after a reasonable length of time. In other words; Patients must not expect to be able to exercise like I have been doing, right from the beginning. Remember that a journey of a thousand miles begins with the first step.

Fortunately, the results of controlled studies on two of the most important issues in the book, give proof that exercise does help to reverse the effects of Pd, and so does the type of medication I took. The other recommendations are all common sense, and we should easily be able to confirmed them as beneficial.

On reflection, I realize that it does not really matter whether I do or don't have Pd. It is purely academic. If all my symptoms are similar to those of other people with Pd, does it matter what name is given to the cause thereof? Does any one of us know for certain that we have Pd and not some other form of Parkinson's? I now know that medical science has come to the conclusion that there are at least four distinctly different forms of Pd. Maybe I am one of those four, or maybe there is a fifth? What really matters is **how we deal with our situation.**

I feel that I do have an obligation to others to tell them what I have been doing successfully, to overcome the effects of most of my Pd symptoms, and if it works on other PwPs, as it has already, then this book serves a very real purpose. The fact that I still have several not-so-obvious symptoms of Pd, is not material at this stage. The medical profession can still sort those problems out, and I can get on with finding the best way to get this book into the homes of every other newly diagnosed PwP throughout the world, which is my objective.

I have regularly visited twelve different support groups, within a sixteen hundred kilometer radius of my home, over the past few years. I am very anxious to find other people who are willing to put the effort into achieving the same results as I have. I want to stress the fact that none of the people at any of these meetings were aware of what I had come to talk to them about. Their reactions to my story, and the thrill they derived from my one-on-one demonstrations of 'How to walk properly by **using the conscious brain**', were completely spontaneous.

The amazing result has been that:

Not one single person, with walking difficulties, regardless of how old or how afflicted, had any problem walking properly, after showing them how to use the conscious brain to control this activity.

On each of my visits, I had made a point of looking very carefully at the people, as they came into the meetings, before I addressed them. In each instance, I was aware of those with walking problems. Everybody present at these meetings witnessed the change in the walking quality of all those who participated.

At my first talk, one man in the small town of Potchefstroom, took a long time to walk, unaided, from the door to his chair, because of his erratic leg movements, which I assumed to have been Dyskinesia. He put up his hand, when I had finished speaking, and asked me if I could show him how to overcome his walking difficulty. I have to be honest and say that I was very reluctant to try my theories out on him, due to the fear of failure. However, if my theory has any value whatsoever, it has to work on everybody. I had to take the bull by the horns.

I first went through the process of asking him, while firmly holding onto his arm, if he was able to stand on his toes? After doing this successfully, I asked him to lift his legs straight up in front of him, one at a time, while flexing his feet. He managed this very easily; better than I could. Lastly I asked him to swing his arms, which he also did. All of these movements he carried out without any problems.

Then I asked him **why he could not perform these actions, when he walked?** He, of course, was unable to answer this question. I explained to him that he was able to do them individually, because he was then using his conscious brain, but when he walks without thinking about it, he uses his subconscious brain, to control his movements.

What I wanted him to do with me was walk, while using his conscious brain, a not-very-easy-to-do task. I told him to concentrate very hard on each movement and not think about anything else. I would be holding his arm firmly, so he could not lose his balance.

We then proceeded to walk together, and while I kept saying "Heel first.... now push forward with the back foot..." etc., **he managed to do it, without any problems whatsoever.** Later, when he walked to the refreshment table, after the meeting, I watched him walk perfectly normally on his own, but then I noticed, he had a huge grin on his face, which spread from ear to ear. He has apparently continued to walk normally ever since, and his doctor has now told him that he does not have Pd. This sounded very familiar.

In Port Shepstone, at my second talk, a lady asked me to show her how to walk, without falling. She battled to stand without someone holding her. She was terribly scared and unsure of herself. She stood with her feet spread fairly well apart, which prompted me to ask the reason why? She explained that she fell over if she did not stand like that. I took hold of her left arm and asked her to stand with her feet together. I explained that, in my opinion, the main reason why she was falling was because her muscles had not got the strength to prevent her from falling, once she started to get off-balance. Also, the Pd adds to the problem by not communicating with the leg muscles in time to initiate the corrective action, needed to avoid falling. I also said that her balance problem was also badly affected by her lack of confidence, which in turn was caused by the memories of previous falls. I said that, with a fair amount of practice, and a lot of physical exercise, to improve muscle strength, she could learn how to consciously control her balance, as I had.

After going through the routine of confirming that she was still able to lift her legs up in front of her, stand on her toes and swing her arms etc, we were soon off around the hall. She was able to walk around the room with me, perfectly normally, while I loosely held her arm and went through the routine of, 'Land on the heel.... push with the back foot.... swing your other arm etc.'. I also told her to keep her shoulders back and her head up, and not to look down on the ground while she was walking. She also had no problem whatsoever, in walking all the way around the hall.

Another man was also keen to try to walk properly, and went through the same routine, with the same result.

Somebody phoned me, on the following Monday morning, when I was back home, and told me that his wife had walked that morning with him on the beach, without any problems, for the first time in many years. He was very excited and emotional at the time and could not thank me enough. I did not make a note of his name or whether it was he who had Pd or his wife. His phone call was all I needed.

At that same Port Shepstone demonstration, there was one man who did not come forward, during the meeting, but approached me at the lunch table afterwards. From memory, he was close to eighty years of age. I had watched him arriving at the hall and had noticed his very slow and tentative progress. He used a three-wheeled walker and had to be assisted to sit down. He asked me if I could show him how to walk. I first of all asked him if he really wanted to start doing physical exercise, at his time of life. I said that he was under no pressure to start learning to walk properly at his age, or to expose himself to the risk of falling. I was worried that he would find that he was physically incapable of walking properly, and land up feeling even more despondent. He spoke with such a faint voice that I could barely hear him.

However, my fears were soon allayed. He was determined to give it a try. I explained the problem that his brain was unable to communicate properly with his legs, with the result that he was unable to walk properly. I further explained that there was nothing actually wrong with his legs, although, the muscles were more or less completely withered, from lack of use. When we got up to give it a try, it was like holding a butterfly on my arm. His first few steps were rather tentative, but before we had reached the end of the table, he was walking quite normally. I could feel all the eyes on us, from around the dining room, and I felt a hush descend over the whole group, because they all knew him well, and knew how badly he walked. When he got back to his seat, he was grinning from ear to ear, and his wife was ecstatic.

Almost immediately afterwards, we were ready to leave the dining room, to go home. We proceeded to walk around a quadrangle, which was under cover, because it had started to rain. This old gentleman was off in front of us with his walker, like a young boy on a scooter. His wife was walking next to me and exclaimed out loud, 'Look at him!' She had not seen him walk like that for a long, long time. It just goes to show that even the most advanced patients can succeed if they set their minds to it.

It has taken me several years to overcome my walking, and other movement difficulties, and therefore I don't expect to see any immediate improvement in other PwP's overall health for some time to come. However, I am very confident, that the condition of some of them can and will improve, if they continue to exercise and adopt a positive attitude.

The question also arises as to whether in fact all the people, who have been able to walk properly with me, by using their conscious brain, have actually got Pd, or whether they possibly have Parkinsonism. Not all PwPs have difficulty walking, or for that matter, eating and drinking, without spilling everything. Perhaps the walking problem is age related and has nothing to do with Pd. I am very aware that older people tend to shuffle, even without Pd.

At the age of fifty-seven, when I was diagnosed, I was not exactly old, and would not have expected to be shuffling, instead of walking. But, I was! That suggests to me that there was another cause, other than age. The photograph on the cover, taken in 2002, does not indicate advanced age. The answer to this question is academic. What matters, is that: -

Millions of people with walking difficulties associated with Pd can now be shown how to walk

properly, by using the conscious brain to control their movements.

They can also be shown how to bring a glass, or a fork, up to the mouth, without spilling the contents.

There is another interesting question. Will all the PwPs with walking difficulties, who have found that they are able to overcome them, have the determination to perfect this new skill, by embarking on a regular walking program? Also: If they regularly do this exercise, will their general health improve to the extent that mine has?

At the time of starting to write about the aftermath of making the contents of this book public, it had been six months since I had seen the neurologist and had stopped taking Eldepryl. During that time, I had kept a diary, in which I recorded all the changes that had taken place in my condition, which I felt were related to Pd, because I felt that it was very important. I do not want to bore you with the actual entries, as I did in the second edition. So I will give you a list of my symptoms, as they occurred:

1. I lost my voice on most days.
2. My emotional state deteriorated noticeably.
3. I experienced coordination problems, while driving
4. I experienced exhaustion again.
5. The supinating worsened, causing pains in my feet and knees.
6. My clumsiness got worse, regularly knocking things over on the dining table.
7. I found that word-finding had deteriorated.
8. My sleeping problems became worse.
9. My hand and leg tremors returned, when waking up.
10. I lost confidence, and found it difficult to negotiate with business people.
11. My hand tremors got worse.
12. My rigidity made it difficult to get out of a chair and stand up straight.
13. My movements, while doing exercises, became jerky again.
14. I have become more irritable and grumpy.
15. I now withdraw into my own world, again.
16. I fall asleep again, during the daytime.
17. I trip, when walking, because of a lack of concentration.

18. I picked up another bad chest infection, which proved very difficult to get rid of.

All these problems slowly disappeared, over the next two years, after going back to walking only three times a week and starting to do special 'Senior Citizen's Fitness Association' gym classes, twice a week. These classes included stretching exercises and movement routines, done to music, which improved muscle coordination.

Since 2007, I have become aware that my self-confidence has improved quite considerably. I am still learning to play bridge, without any apprehension, although I have found great difficulty in remembering what suit is trumps and what cards have been played. I have also started to do art again, and am enjoying it very much. We now live in a retirement village and I occasionally sing to the residents, at special functions. I do still have a few problems with word finding, but my confidence is much improved in this area

Part 5

Warning

I want to caution you against any false optimism. Whatever benefit you stand to derive, will be entirely dependent upon the effort you are prepared to invest in your own physical and mental fitness; nothing more, and nothing less!

If you are unable to walk at all, or else you are too rigid to be able to do any meaningful exercise, then be very cautious. However, I have had the experience of working with two patients, who were wheelchair bound. Both of whom were able to walk properly, when concentrating on their actions.

Your age may possibly be against changing your lifestyle.

You may be suffering from severe side effects of medication, about which you are not able to do anything.

You may not have the patience to do all the things I recommend, before giving up. You are human!

Please don't think this warning means I don't think anybody will benefit from this book. I definitely do not think this. I have had many emails, telling me how much benefit people have had from reading my book. See some in Appendix 2.

I obviously cannot lay claim that, because _I_ have been able to overcome many of the symptoms of Pd, every other Person with Pd, or maybe Parkinsonism, will be able to do the same.

Think about what I have said in the book and make your own decision, as to whether you have faith in it or not.

If you do decide to make a change to your lifestyle, then don't expect miracles overnight. Bodily fitness will improve all the while you continue to do energetic exercise, until it reaches a natural level, commensurate with your age and medical condition. Your physical health and your mental health go hand in hand. When you become more positive about yourself, and your muscles and joints are being used properly, and your body is becoming more fit and healthy; then you will feel the benefit of your efforts. If, however, you give it all a half-hearted shot, to see what will happen, then you will be sadly disappointed, and you will feel let-down. Rather give it your best shot, stick to it, and you will derive a great deal of benefit from your efforts.

Part 6

Conclusion

Yes, **it is possible to reverse the effects of Pd.** How well you manage to achieve this, will depend entirely upon your attitude; how much you are prepared to commit yourself to regular **energetic** exercise; whether you are able to persuade your doctor to prescribe Azilect; how positive you are and how successful you are in managing your harmful stress levels.

The Question Still Is: Do I really have Pd?

This is a perplexing question. I can only set out the facts, and you have to draw your own conclusion. **I have no doubt whatsoever that I do still have Pd,** for the following reasons:

- Two eminently qualified neurologists diagnosed my Pd.
- I took a potent Pd medication for ten years. If I did not have Pd, then this would have had serious effects on me.
- My knowledge of the intricacies of Pd could only have been obtained by study, or having Pd. I have never studied any form of medicine. It stands to reason that I must have Pd.
- I wrote my book claiming: I thought regular energetic exercise had helped me to overcome the debilitating effects of many of my Pd symptoms, long before proof of this claim was found. Scientifically controlled double blind studies, have been carried out by the University of Pennsylvania, the University of Southern California and the University of Frankfurt, showing that certain types of regular energetic exercise produce Glial Derived Neurotrophic Factor (GDNF) in the brain, which repairs damaged brain cells, and slows down or even reverses the progression of Pd. This *has* happened to me.
- I took part in a regimen of regular energetic exercise, long before I was finally diagnosed with Pd. Because of this exercise, I have assumed that this was the reason why it took over twenty-five years, after my first Pd symptoms first presented themselves, before my Pd was diagnosed
- I also stated, in that book, that the manufacturers of Eldepryl claimed their medication could slow down or even reverse the progression of Pd, long before the news of a

119

seven-year double blind scientifically controlled study, confirming this claim was released. This has also appeared to have been true in my case.

- My symptoms only started to improve after I started taking Eldepryl. Since taking the Eldepryl, I have found that my condition got worse, when I stopped the medication, even though I continued the exercise. Likewise, when I stopped the exercise, my condition also deteriorated, even though I was still taking the medication.

- My personal discovery of the way to **consciously control my movements, enabling me to walk normally and bring food and drink to my mouth successfully, have all worked on everybody, to whom I have demonstrated this methodology.** How else would I have known this?

- The fact that: my methods of teaching PwP's how to walk properly and successfully; get food and drink into the mouth; are currently used by speech therapists to help patients to speak with facial expression. This must prove that this is an established approach to treatment. I had not been aware of this, when I discovered it for myself, in the late 1990's

- My list of symptoms could not possibly be for anything other than Pd – see Appendix 1.

Opposition to the Sale of This Book

As stated earlier in this chapter, two senior neurologists took the trouble to come to an AGM, after I was asked to stand down as Chairman, and after I had been asked to resign from the PASA committee. This could mean that they were very intent on persuading me, and the local Parkinson's community, that what I had said in my book, would mislead patients, and cause them more problems than they already had. It could also possibly mean that I presented a threat to neurologists, if more patients started to improve. I will give them the benefit of the doubt, at this stage.

As far as PASA is concerned, their motivation is very doubtful indeed. They had proof copies of the book, long before that AGM. So, why did they not speak to me about their concerns, instead of clandestinely attacking me at the AGM? They did not give notice of their intention to make a prepared statement at that meeting, nor did they advise members of the impending attendance, at that meeting, of the two neurologists. In addition to these two oversights, they made no mention of this fiasco in the minutes of that AGM, and when the members refused to approve those minutes at the next AGM, they still refused to make mention of those events, and the committee irregularly approved those minutes, at their next meeting.

This all smells of a bit of skullduggery, but at whose instigation, I do not know. Let it suffice to say that if there is a genuine concern about my book, having a possible harmful effect on patients, then I would have thought that there would have been a better way of going about dealing with it. At present, the only opposition to my activities, comes from PASA and some neurologists, who state quite categorically that I do not have Pd. As this is only hearsay, I have to ignore it, but if my story of having Pd is correct, as I believe it is, then how can they say this, without having examined me?

My final question is:

Now that we know that, taking an MAO-B inhibitor and doing regular energetic exercise, can both slow down, or even reverse Pd symptoms, then why don't neurologists pass all this knowledge on to their patients, with movement disorders, when they make the diagnosis?

My final statement to you is:

Too much *reliance* on medication alone, can reduce our chances of enjoying a better quality of life. We must therefore take full control of our lives, and enjoy the benefits that will follow from the taking of the most suitable medication and living a healthier lifestyle.

Recommendations

To finish off this story of hope and encouragement, I would like to reiterate eleven steps you need to take, to help maximize your chances of living a progressively fuller and more rewarding life. Although Pd is a degenerative disease, and its prognosis is not very good, *there is no reason to adopt a negative attitude,* from the very onset of the disease.

It has been proven that exercise definitely improves our quality of life, and **it cannot do us any harm,** if we do it properly, under advice from a qualified person.

I also believe that, if your body becomes less rigid and more flexible, and you are able to treat the disease as a challenge, then your condition **CAN** improve, and then you **WILL** progressively feel a lot better.

At worst, I believe that if, in some cases, the progression of Pd may not be halted, it, at least, can be retarded.

How To Set About Improving Your Condition

1. Get rid of anything that causes *negative stress.* This includes coming to terms with any unresolved *trauma,* which still exists in your life.

At the time of diagnosis, were you in a great deal of stress, or had you had something traumatic happen to you, immediately preceding the diagnosis? Most PwP's have difficulty handling stress. Many express a desire to learn more about the management of stress. There are many books available in libraries and bookstores, and I strongly recommend that you read as much about it as possible. Harmful stress occurs on a regular basis. It is not something you can permanently put behind you. Every time you realize that you are getting harmfully stressed, analyze the cause of the stress, and take immediate steps to remove that cause. Then take steps to see that it does not happen again, if that is possible. This may seem a little idealistic, but it really isn't. Most of my harmful stress comes from my dealings with other people. When I go over each stress situation, I invariably find that **I am the problem,** and have had to change many of my attitudes, in order to avoid future stressful situations arising. I often assume that everybody knows all about Pd, while in reality, few people know anything at all about the disease. Have patience with other people, talk openly about your problems, and help others to understand your situation.

The way that I learned to reduce my stress at work was to make a **list, every morning**, of all the things I had to do each day. I then numbered each task, in order of importance. Then, as the day moved on, I marked off all the tasks I had completed, before proceeding with the next most urgent task. Sometimes, I got through all the tasks, but invariably I didn't, because I never knew what new problems would hit my desk during the course of each day. Because I knew, from experience, that other problems were bound to appear, without any warning, I should have made allowances for this, and given myself more time, but I never did. Don't try to cram too much into any one-day, because that is how we create stress for ourselves.

2. Learn how to eat healthily, and in *moderation*.

If, like me, you are not thin, eating in excess of our needs, puts on weight and puts more strain on our muscles and joints. We should therefore endeavor to regulate our intake of the wrong types of food. I cannot lecture on this subject! I am very fond of my food, and admit to regularly eating too much.

If you are underweight, then you should try to eat more, and more often, and try to make the food more palatable. You need to eat fruit and vegetables, to get all the nutrients and vitamins your body requires. You should avoid eating protein, within an hour before or after taking medication containing levodopa. Get into the habit of weighing yourself at regular intervals, and keeping a note of the results. It is easier to lose or gain weight, if you have a goal to work towards.

3. Establish a daily energetic exercise program.

This is the most important task of all. Exercise and Pd, do not go comfortably hand-in-hand. It is a habit, which requires a great deal of effort to cultivate, especially if you have not done regular exercise for many years. When I talk about walking, I don't mean taking the dog for a stroll. That falls under the heading of relaxation. Walking, must involve a reasonable amount of exertion, and the pulse rate should be elevated above one hundred beats per minute, and held there for at least twenty minutes. This cannot be achieved at the beginning, but should be part of your goal. When you start your program, you would be ill advised to exceed more than ten minutes walking, **every second day,** for the first two weeks, and then increase that by five minutes, every **second** week, if you can. You should also aim to increase your effort all the time, by setting regular goals, and keeping records of your achievements. If you manage to walk one kilometer in ten minutes, when you start; that should improve, both in distance and time, until you are walking possibly six kilometers in an hour. Don't forget; **before you walk, you should do some loosening-up** and **stretching exercises,** and **afterwards, you should do some more stretching exercises**.

Your physiotherapist will help you with all these exercises. Don't be foolish and think that you don't need to warm-up and stretch before or afterwards. Because of your inherent rigidity, you will need these more than anyone else, and if you don't do them, you will almost certainly pick up injuries. **Do NOT do strenuous exercise every day.** Your body needs to have a day for recovery, after any prolonged exercise. If you do not heed this warning, your muscles will not have time to recover and they will stand a good chance of becoming injured. I personally now walk three times a week, for a total of twenty-four kilometers. I also go, twice a week for an hour, to special gym classes for senior citizens.

4. Find ways you enjoy stimulating your brain.

This is the fun part of the 'apparent recovery' process. Some of us tend to sideline our brains, as we get older; offering excuses for not wanting to learn anything new; saying that we are too old to learn, when we really mean that we **don't want to make fools of ourselves**. Put your pride in your pocket, and get out there, and learn how to play bridge or canasta. Alternatively, learn to use a computer, or to play a musical instrument, or surf the Internet. Any activity, which uses the brain rather than the body, can be very stimulating. Remember, it is your brain, which is the problem, not your body, and anything you can do to stimulate the brain is good. It is all well and good being active occasionally, but you have to learn to fill all your days with enjoyable activities.

5. Adopt a positive attitude.

Have you ever experienced the joy of meeting someone, who exudes energy and good vibes? These people are no different to us. They all have problems; bills to pay and deadlines to meet. What makes them different? Simple! They have a **positive attitude**. None of us is positive all the time. We all go through periods of negativity, but they snap out it very quickly, because they find it very destructive. Why be negative? **Our attitude determines the outcome of everything we do.** It also affects everybody, with whom we come into contact. Think of the positive results you will enjoy, in your interpersonal relationships. People will always be happy to be with you, even though you have Pd. Remember, attitudes are the determining factor in relationships, and especially in conflict situations. Attitude is akin to the spice we put into our food. Without it, the food would still be wholesome and nutritious, but it would not taste the same. When a good deed is done with the wrong attitude, it can appear to be anything but a good deed. Try to be, as you would like others to be. The best way to make a change in your relationships is to **take a good hard look at *your own* attitudes.** When you point a finger at others, take a good look at where all the other fingers are pointing. Wherever there is conflict, there is seldom a completely innocent party. The blame can usually be attributed to both sides, and often, more towards oneself than the other party. You will never develop, as a person, if you don't accept responsibility for your own actions. Blaming others, for your failures, will only alienate their feelings towards you, and diminish your credibility. Being positive, is not just an attitude; **it is a way of life.** You can choose to be positive or negative.

There is nothing to beat being POSITIVE!

6.   Adjust your *physical* and *mental activities,* to suit your prevailing health situation.

Our state of health is not always the same from day to day, or even from minute to minute. We cannot *expect* to feel the same, all the time, and we therefore have to adjust our activities to suit the way we feel now. It is no good pretending to be gung-ho, when we feel terrible. We will not fool anyone. We have to adjust our activities to suit the way we feel.

7.   Develop the habit of remaining *active* in the daytime.

I find great pleasure in reading and listening to music, but I am aware that these activities must not take up a disproportionate amount of my time, and become an impediment to my overall health. I cannot explain this, but I know it makes me lethargic. This type of activity must be reserved for the time we have left, after we have dealt with our other more strenuous activities. There are always jobs to be done around the house and garden, unless you are one, who hates manual labor. If you have this problem, then there is always a need for people to help others, doing charitable work.

8.   Perform troublesome movements differently, by using your *conscious* brain. Help your brain bypass

the *Pd effect,* by finding other ways of performing them.

This is probably the most exciting part of the 'apparent recovery' process. Don't give in when you keep dropping things, knocking objects over, or are generally being clumsy. Take a step back, and think about what you have just done, and then go through it all again, only this time, concentrating hard on what you're doing. You will find that you don't drop things when you concentrate hard on what you're doing. Accidents happen, when you allow your mind to wander. When that happens, you revert to the subconscious brain, to control your movements. There is nothing you cannot do by using your conscious brain, providing of course that there is nothing else physically wrong with you. Use a little bit of ingenuity. Get **into the habit of laughing, when something goes wrong**. Others might not find it easy to laugh, when you break something valuable. Help them to see things in the light of **your** knowledge of Pd. Get into the habit of not touching valuable objects, just in case your mind gets distracted, and you have an accident.

9.   Take an active interest in your medication

Read every slip contained in the medication package, and assure yourself that you have no inherent problem with that medication. You may have been taking it for years, not knowing that there is a contra-indication on that slip, because of some other condition you have, or some other medication you take. If you think that you are taking too much, or too little medication, or you feel that it is not doing you any good, then talk to your doctor. He or she is there to help you, and relies a lot on your feedback. Always try to be part of the solution, and not part of the problem.

If you are lucky enough to be taking Azilect, and you are able to tolerate it; and you also take levodopa medication, you should expect to take less levodopa medication. Otherwise, you may develop dyskinesia, which is a sign of having too much dopamine in the brain.

10.   Learn how to deal with new symptoms.

If you feel a new symptom, starting to make its presence felt in your life, then examine it carefully and get to know exactly how it affects you. Then pass this knowledge on to your doctor. When you get to know how each symptom affects you, then you will be able to see if you can do anything to overcome its effects. Don't be negative. Try to see it as one more challenge. When all else fails, and you have not managed to overcome the problem, then make up your mind that it is not going to get you down. Get used to it and forget about it.

Pacing Yourself

The following checklist comes in handy, when assessing whether or not you are pacing yourself properly.

- You must continually take steps to keep all *negative stress* under control.
- Continually watch your intake of food, and alcohol.
- Take an *active* interest in your *medication.*
- Continually keep your brain *stimulated.*
- Continually examine your *attitude* towards others.
- Look for ways to *consciously overcome* any new Pd related symptoms.
- Stay Positive

All of these facts tell me that, **taking an MAO-B inhibitor** and **doing regular energetic exercise**, is the only way to bring about an improvement in Pd. The other factors of:

- **Managing harmful stress levels,**
- **Adopting a positive attitude**
- **Participating in regular 'brain exercises'**

have all helped me to achieve my current good health and can only be good for all of us.

There is no way on earth that I can guarantee your success, if you do decide to set about trying to do what I have done, but I hope that you will try and give it your best shot.

Whoever you are, there is nothing to be lost, and everything to be gained, by following these simple rules, listed above.

I wish you all the very best of health for the future, and hope that you will *treat Pd as a challenge,* and not a "virtual death sentence".

YOUR health is in *YOUR* hands, so why not take full control of it, NOW?

Appendix 1
Details of My Symptoms

In order to dispel any doubts about my claim to be a PwP, I feel compelled to give you a complete list of all the Pd related health problems, at the time of being diagnosed, and subsequently. Most of the problems are symptoms of Pd, or problems related to Pd. Others are possibly caused by medication.

This list will also help some readers to derive a little bit of comfort from the knowledge that they are not alone in some of their experiences. We all experience a reluctance to tell others about little health problems, which happen to us from time to time, and the odd ache or pain we experience, believing them to be inconsequential. I have often accepted certain problems without question, believing them to be some quirk of nature, which happens every now and then, to all of us, like getting a "stitch", when we ran around as children.

However, it is surprising how many problems are actually symptoms of this peculiar disorder. Because of my lack of knowledge about Pd, many of my symptoms were not recognized by me, or the neurologist, at the time of diagnosis in 1992

The account of my 'apparent recovery' from a lot of these symptoms is what I want to dwell upon, and unless you know what my symptoms were in the first place, it would be difficult to know, and understand, the whole story.

The symptoms are listed in alphabetical order. There is no intention of classifying them in any order of importance. A lot of time has elapsed, since I first presented with these symptoms, therefore the timing of arrival may be a little inaccurate. Where the symptom is still present, I talk about it in the present tense. Those that are no longer present, I talk about in the past tense.

Please take note that, not all of these symptoms, listed below are necessarily regarded, by the medical profession, as those of Parkinson's disease. However, I have listed all the irregularities that have happened to me, since the Pd started, and which, I feel, are connected to a brain problem.

Bad Posture and Limping

During the late eighties, Shirley asked me why I was walking so badly, when we were together, in one of the local shopping malls. I had no idea what she was talking about. She also said that I looked as if I were limping.

Soon after that, this bad posture did come to my attention, when I was on my way to the gymnasium, early one morning. The sun was low above the horizon, casting a long shadow on the ground, which showed quite clearly that I was noticeably leaning forward at the hips. This gave me quite a shock. To me, the shadow looked like that of an old man, but I was, in my mind, still young, and the shock of seeing myself walking so badly, for no apparent reason, gave my self-confidence a bigger knock than the limping had. Was this 'normal'? Was I really becoming an old man, already?

After Diagnosis, when I had taken stock of myself, I found that my shoulders were hunched forward, and the left was lower than the right, which meant that my head was leaning to the left. I was not swinging my right arm, which I held firmly against my waist, with the forearm parallel to the ground, as if I were holding something in my hand. The right thumb was held rigidly at a right angle to my hand, and my fingers were tented. Although, when I became aware of it, I was able to consciously move it down to my side, and swing it.

My stride was quite short, which is surprising for someone who is over one-comma-eight meters (six feet) tall. I appeared to walk with a limp, although there was no obvious reason for this. I was not injured, nor was one leg shorter than the other. I have managed to overcome this problem by controlling my walk and using my conscious brain, to control my movement. When I am not concentrating on my walking, it still reverts back to the shuffle and limp.

Biting the Inside of My Mouth and Tongue

This may not be a symptom of Pd, although I have spoken to many people about it and it appears to be very common amongst PwPs. It also seems to be quite logical, as it involves the muscles in the tongue, lips and cheeks, which help to move food around in the mouth, while chewing. If these movements are not coordinated properly, they are bound to get in the way of the teeth, while the jaw is closing. The right-hand side of the inside of my lower lip, and both inner cheeks, bear the scars. It appears to happen in cycles.

The scar, on the inside of my lower right lip, is dead in line with the right eyeteeth, and the scars, on the inside of my cheeks, are in line with the back molars.

Clumsiness

I have been getting progressively clumsier, over the past few years. The awkwardness is not confined to walking over uneven surfaces, but also occurs, when climbing up stairs, when I continually trip, and not only when they are of unequal height. I think I do not lift my knees sufficiently.

The acts of eating and drinking became a bit of a nightmare to me. The number of times I have knocked items over, on the dinner table, has become legend in my family. At one stage, spilling my food became so embarrassing, that I was reluctant to eat in up-market restaurants any more.

Another example, of my clumsiness, is more closely related to inter-personal activities. Ever since my years as a teenager, I had always enjoyed ballroom dancing, and prided myself on my dancing ability. As the Pd started to assert itself, my skills on the dance floor, slowly vanished. Now, not even Shirley gets any pleasure being pushed around by her clumsy husband.

Dropping things has generally never appeared to be a problem, other than my food, while putting it into my mouth. However, I have become well known for knocking over crockery and glasses at the dinner table. My hands seem to take a circuitous route to, or from the intended object. They do not appear to go directly to or from that object. They take a route, which defies logic. The objects, which I regularly knock over, are never directly in the path, which my hand would be expected to take. I cannot explain this problem. Dragging utensils onto my lap is another common occurrence. It always leaves me flabbergasted, when these things happen. My reaction afterwards is always, "How did that happen?" It appears that I do not let go of the glass or cup, consequently, dragging it back towards me.

I regularly bruise myself, bumping into furniture, doorknobs and doorjambs. I seem to have so many things to think about, when I am walking, that I don't seem to take too much notice of obstacles in my path.

Confusion with left and right sides

I have never before had a problem knowing my left from my right. However, now, I have to think very carefully, because my immediate action is to go right, when I should go left. I know others also suffer from this, but there has to be a reason for it.

Constipation

Even as a child, this was a problem. It may have had something to do with spending long hours in air-raid shelters, where we had no toilet facilities, and when it was too dangerous to go outside. It is not surprising, therefore, that I did not take too much notice of this problem. As a young adult, I had never had a regular bowel motion, but in the early eighties, long before diagnosis, it became appreciably worse.

I lived on patent remedies, which were mostly based on the Senna plant. This could have caused a lot of damage, had it not been for 'Lactose intolerance, which required an internal examination. The lactose intolerance started in the early seventies. The specialist told me I had to introduce a more natural means of keeping my bowels regular. He advised a fiber-rich diet, accompanied by a regular intake of fresh and dried fruit. Shirley and I were already in the habit of eating a lot of vegetables and fresh fruit, so the addition of dried fruit was a pleasure, especially when mixed with the cooked food.

The new diet worked well, for a while, but I needed to vary it, so that I did not eat dried fruit every day, otherwise it did not work regularly. Excuse the pun! I typically try to have dried fruit one day, a dish with onions and/or garlic the next, and a meal devoid of either on the third day. This was not a fixed routine, but when I missed a day without a bowel motion, all I had to do was eat some fruit cake or dried apricots, or some dish with onions, to do the trick. When I cannot do any walking, the constipation definitely gets worse.

Depression

It is impossible to establish when I was first diagnosed with severe depression, because our family doctor, from those days, no longer has these records. What I do remember is that it was around the time I moved my factory to Johannesburg.

At the time this problem raised its ugly head, my doctor put me on anti-depressant tablets, which I took for periods of a month or two at a time. I carried on taking anti depressants, on and off for a few years. Later on, in the late eighties, when it started to get worse, my current doctor referred me to a psychologist, for further investigation. After several visits to this very pleasant young man, he was at a complete loss to even begin to understand why I had this problem. I had no hang-ups about anything. I had no unresolved problems, no trouble at home, nothing worrying me at work, other than my overwhelming workload, and my concerns about the political and social problems in South Africa. He thought that my workload was a problem, but it was not responsible for my depression, because even though I worked long hours, I enjoyed my work to the full. It was a challenge, and I enjoyed a challenge. As far as the political and social problems were concerned, he pointed out that they were something over which I had no control, and if I could not come to terms with them, then I should seriously consider leaving the country.

Depression was the most debilitating symptom, because it **robbed me of the will to help myself**. It made me feel beaten, and took away my natural desire to fight for survival.

Difficulty Swallowing and choking

This problem did not happen too often in the beginning, but now it happens very frequently. When it does happen, it causes a considerable amount of discomfort and anxiety.

In my case, the choking seems to be caused by food, or saliva, dropping off the back of my tongue and into my open windpipe. At least, this is how I have described it to my neurologist. The food, apparently, does not get gathered together properly, by the tongue, before it is swallowed; or else by a saliva build-up in the mouth. Fortunately, it has never been life threatening, but it is always uncomfortable and frightening, not just to me but to my family as well. This is not confined to food alone. It more frequently happens with liquids, especially vinegar, on which I have nearly choked on many occasions.

There are other problems, related to swallowing. I am unable to swallow certain food items, such as various forms of potatoes, either boiled, baked, roasted, mashed or even French fries. The list is not solely confined to potatoes. Bread and meat are also major culprits. All the food items, which have given me problems, have one characteristic in common; they are all dry. There is not enough saliva in the mouth or throat, to allow the food to travel all the way down to the stomach, with the result that it sticks in my throat and I choke, or it sticks further down, before entering the stomach. Then I am unable to swallow anything. I get hiccups and a very uncomfortable feeling in my chest.. The choking could be very dangerous, but I am usually able to sense when it is happening, because the food seems to stick to my tongue; so I take a drink of water, to wash the food down.

Dribbling

Dribbling is a symptom that is very degrading, akin almost to being incontinent. It has made me feel like a baby again; unable to control my bodily functions.

This, fortunately, mainly happened while sleeping. When I awoke in the mornings, there would be a big wet patch of saliva on the pillow: an unwelcome reminder of my new status in life. I am not aware of dribbling at any other time, although my daughter has mentioned that I sometimes dribbled at the dinner table.

When I became aware of the dribbling, I merely had to close my mouth and swallow. The lack of swallowing is the cause of the dribbling. Because I have a nasal blockage, I often can't breathe easily, through my nose, with the result that I often breathe through the mouth. So, when breathing through the mouth, while eating, I was not swallowing the excess saliva, and it was running out of the open mouth.

Dry Mouth

The dry mouth *can* occur as a side effect of medication, although I have often heard it referred to as a symptom of Pd, when I have attended seminars.

Sometimes, I have felt that the dry mouth is possibly caused by stress, because it often happens when I am in a stressful situation. However, it does not *always* happen that way, as it has happened, when I am enjoying myself, with my family.

It also happens, when I find myself breathing through my mouth, instead of my nose. There is no reason for this, other than sometimes, but not always, having constricted nasal passages. It could possibly be medication related but, as I do not often make changes to my medication, it is unlikely.

Falling Asleep During the Daytime

Whether my lack of sleep, during the night, was the cause of my falling asleep during the daytime, I do not know. This phenomenon only started to occur during the eighties, after more than fifteen years of being able to sleep less than four hours a night.

I started to fall asleep at my desk, without being aware that I was even feeling sleepy. I occasionally found my head suddenly falling down onto the keyboard of my computer. Not only was this embarrassing, in front of my staff, but it was worrying. I have to admit that the screen of a computer can cause me to become a bit mesmerized, especially after many uninterrupted hours of working.

Driving my car did not escape this problem either. Fortunately for me, I seldom, if ever, travel further than a few kilometers on my own. I normally have Shirley with me, and she watches me like a hawk. There were a few occasions when she could see that my gaze was becoming fixed and glassy. On each of those occasions she would speak to me, which immediately diffused the situation. That was, other than once, when I was approaching a robot (Traffic light), at the end of an off-ramp, after having driven for over an hour on the freeway. The car was almost at the stop when, without warning, I fell asleep. Shirley shouted at me and I was able to complete the stop without any incident.

When I am driving now, and begin to feel my eyes closing I always stop and either change drivers, or have a break.

This phenomenon does not appear to be related to tiredness, but rather to my state of mind. It has the potential to be very dangerous. Many patients with Pd have stopped driving for this reason.

Fatigue

In my case, fatigue is something, which I would normally have expected. Not because I thought I worked too much, but because I knew that I didn't sleep enough. This fatigue only started to happen during the eighties, long after I had developed the habit of sleeping for less than half the normally recommended time. It manifested itself in several ways. I had periods of time when I felt incredibly tired, and yet I battled to sleep. During these periods of fatigue, I was listless and lacked energy, even when I had just woken up. The fatigue was often accompanied by spasms of yawning, when my eyes watered profusely. This still happens to this day (2010). The only way I have found to get out of this lassitude was to do something energetic, like walking, although, getting started was sometimes very difficult. Walking invariably did the trick, and it also helped me to sleep better.

Another sign, of possible exhaustion, was that I often fell asleep in the company of visitors, especially at the dinner table, although I was never really aware of this. Shirley allowed me to sleep, wherever I was, while often having to apologize to guests for my bad behavior. When she told me afterwards, that I had been sleeping, I usually denied it, saying that I only had my eyes closed, but claimed to be listening to what was going on. Whether I was really asleep, or not, didn't really matter. I was not behaving normally. This may be more to do with one of the previous symptoms.

There are times when I am completely sapped of all energy, and find it difficult to hold my head upright, on my shoulders. This feeling, of total exhaustion, comes on without warning, and usually, when I am relaxing.

Flexed Calves, When Sitting

I notice, while I am sitting at my computer or watching television that my right heel, and sometimes the left, is always up in the air. There is no reason for this, other than possibly a bad habit, but I don't think so. I am sure it has something to do with Parkinson's, or maybe Dystonia. Nobody in their right mind would sit with the feet on tip-toe.

Flexed Toes When Driving

This is probably not Parkinson's either, but a Dystonia symptom. I am only aware of this happening, while I am driving. The toes on both feet, but more so on the right, curl up tightly. This foot is the one on the accelerator. When I become conscious of it, I am able to consciously relax the toes, but they soon curl up tightly again, within minutes.

Foot Cramps

When in bed, mostly while I am awake, I often get various cramps, in either foot; my right foot, more often than not. It is easy to initiate the cramp, at any time, by turning my right foot to the left, with the toes curled downwards, as far as possible.

To overcome these cramps, I have to pull the foot upwards in a flexed position, usually with the other foot, because I battle to touch my toes with either hand, and especially not with both hands. It also sometimes happens in my sleep, but I don't recall what muscles are involved, but in each case, I have to pull the foot upwards to get the cramped muscle to relax. These cramps, like most, are very painful. Whilst in bed, I don't do anything to cause the cramps, they just happen.

I am now under the impression that this is a Dystonia symptom, also, but it seems to be fairly common among Pd patients.

Frequent Night-time Urination

This problem is normally associated with sugar diabetes. Therefore, I have had my sugar checked on several occasions, and every test has proved negative.

I do not understand what causes the problem, but I am assured that it is Pd related. What brought this problem on was a mystery to me. Why does it not happen all the time? Occasionally, when I suffered from a dry mouth, during the daytime and consequently drank a lot of water, I knew that I was going to get very little sleep that night, because I would be paying several visits to the bathroom. The dry mouth is not *always* a precursor to the urination problem.

I do not understand why the increase in frequency, happens mainly at nighttime? I have to urinate as often as eight times, within a three-hour period.

Frequent Urges to Urinate

Often, when I get the urge to urinate, I get to the toilet and I can't pass any water at all. I have to be careful about this, because, when it is the real thing, and I think the urge will pass, as it often does, I land up wetting myself. I often get this sudden urge, when driving, which makes life very awkward. It often happens in the kitchen or bathroom.

It never occurred to me to question this phenomenon, even though I should have realized that, it was not normal.

Hands Freezing in a Flexed Position

As I have already mentioned, with the carrying of the suitcases: using my hands to perform the odd manual tasks, it started to become a real problem during the eighties. When performing tasks, such as carrying a case, or using a screwdriver, to fasten a screw, my right hand would freeze in the working position and then the shaking would start.

Being right-handed; in order to release my hand, when the freezing took place, I needed to use my left hand to prize the hand open. I suppose that if I had waited a while, for my hand to relax, it would have rectified itself, but I never had the patience to do that.

I noticed that the hand went completely white, where it touched the case handle or screwdriver, and the surrounding flesh went bright red. This does not normally happen to my hand, when I use it. It is not uncommon for hands to show marks, where pressure is applied to them, but my hands show very exaggerated white marks, where contact was made, surrounded by deep red marks. These marks take a time to disappear, when I let go, which I don't think is normal.

Inability to Concentrate

Whether or not this is a recognized Parkinson's symptom, I do not know. What I do know is that, although I was often told at school that I did not concentrate, I have never battled to concentrate on matters that interested me.

This may signify that I am very shallow, or maybe that I exhibit selfish traits, but I need to be as forthright as possible, when talking about these symptoms.

The lack of concentration also affects my walking, when I have to concentrate on the actual movement. Fortunately, the resultant awkwardness, makes me aware of the lapse in concentration.

Long before I was diagnosed, I became quite perturbed by the frequency of periods, when writing programs, that I could not concentrate on what I was doing. This is not typical of my behavior. I am normally very focused, especially when it is something as important as programming. I have been known to be entirely unaware of my surroundings, during this time, and to go for excessively long periods between having something to drink or eat. Shirley tells me that I would perish if I did not have someone looking after me.

Inability to Handle Conflict Situations

Handling conflict situations has become quite a problem in my life, and I therefore avoid them like the plague. When I have not been able to avoid a conflict, since the seventies, I have invariably acted rather irrationally. I have been unable to handle these situations, without getting the shakes, raising my voice and gesticulating with my hands. When I say, "Conflict Situations" I don't mean major rows, I mean anything, from a mild set-to on the telephone, with someone who is reluctant to pay his account, to a mild dressing down from Shirley, because I have forgotten to phone her, when I knew I was going to be home late from work. None of these situations could be described as a major conflict, but they are enough to send me into a complete tailspin. I get the shakes, lose my voice, jump up and down like a jack-in-the-box; and become very abrasive, which does not do my personal relationships any good.

These incidents have become a major stumbling block in my life. I have to learn to let them wash right over me, as if nothing abnormal has happened, otherwise I will not be able to carry on.

Inability to Maintain Balance

Walking in a straight line, or balancing on one leg, is not something we do often. Normally we associate this activity with the need to prove to our friends that we are not under the influence of alcohol, especially at a party.

There must be many stories about PwPs, who have been apprehended, while driving a car, and being unable to convince the law officer, that he or she is not under the influence of alcohol. This applies, not only to balance, but to speech as well.

Balance is often very important indeed, especially when dressing and undressing. Of course, there are other ways of dressing, which don't require us to stand on one leg. However, having done so, since childhood, changing those habits has proved rather difficult. I am not a creature of habit, other than dressing, when I invariably do it the same way every day. Because I didn't think I needed to change my modus operandi, I have had many near falls in my bedroom.

Only after I had been diagnosed, did I make allowances for my condition, but then, only when I thought about it, otherwise, I carry on doing it in the same old way.

When we need our balance most, is while we are walking, especially on uneven surfaces. None of us older people like to fall. So, like most people of my age, I had the odd occasion, when I lost my balance, and either fell, or more often, just managed to save myself. I did not ever get seriously hurt, but I always managed to give myself a fright.

At this point, I must mention my Meniere's Syndrome. I am not too sure whether I really do have Meniere's; the jury is still out on that one. Even the specialist E.N.T.s, have not been sure. All I know is that I have this continual tinnitus in my left ear, and every now and then, I get quite giddy, and have to sit or lie down. Balance is also a Pd problem, and whether mine is the one or the other is purely academic at this stage.

Inability to Manipulate My Fingers

Fastening small buttons on my shirt, started to become difficult during the eighties, as did anything else requiring delicate manipulation.

The muscles in my arms and hands behaved as if they were very cold. I could not get my fingers to do anything; they simply would not react to what I was telling them to do. Muscles don't work very well, when they are very cold, but this sensation, had nothing to do with temperature. I found that I had no real control over my fingers at all, they simply would not move, when and where I wanted. Sometimes, this experience felt worse than others. When muscles are very cold, they still move, but very sluggishly.

The problem had nothing to do with the tremor. The lack of control of my muscles was obviously brought about by the problem of getting the message from the brain to the fingers. The lack of muscle control combined with the tremor; only made life more difficult for me.

Inability to Multi-task

Driving my car, since the early nineties, has become a bit of a problem. I found that it has become difficult to perform two different tasks, simultaneously, particularly when I am in heavy traffic. Tasks such as, changing gear, working the clutch, and indicating while turning a corner, all at the same time, invariably got my pulse racing. The ladies will say that this has nothing to do with Pd either. It is just because I am a man! What do I expect?

Similarly, I cannot successfully hold more than one object in any one hand, at the same time, without eventually dropping one of them. For instance; when carrying objects out of the car, I invariably pick up the various bits and pieces, using all available fingers and thumbs, while conveniently holding the car keys, between my right thumb and forefinger. The moment I try to use the keys, to lock the car door, everything else being held in my right hand, invariably falls to the ground. I cannot control the fingers, in the way, to which, I have always been accustomed. This may seem like an insignificant problem to most people, but to me, it is one more nail in the coffin. Every time I drop something, it robs me of a bit more of my self-confidence.

Inability to Walk on Uneven Surfaces

Going back again to the seventies, I became aware that, walking over uneven surfaces, caused me to feel very clumsy, awkward and insecure. While walking, I found it very difficult to avoid stumbling, when the ground, which I was stepping onto, was lower, or tripping, when it was higher. Both of these results caused painful jolting, which only exacerbated the problem in my lower back.

This first came to my notice, while crossing the playing fields, during those visits to my son's school, to watch him playing rugby. Again, I thought this had something to do with my back problems, and therefore did nothing about it.

When I was younger, I was much more agile, having no problem at all navigating rough ground, rocks and obstacles. I had become like an old man, needing someone to hold onto, while walking on, what looked suspiciously like, flat ground.

Inability to Write Properly

I had already become aware that writing was very problematic during the late sixties, many years before being diagnosed. Although I was able to write very legibly, at the start, my writing quickly deteriorated into a scrawl, which soon became a meaningless squiggle, not even I could understand. I was not aware, at that time, that it also got smaller and smaller. I only realized this when the neurologist pointed it out to me.

At the time I became aware of the writing problem, one of my daily tasks was to make out Work Instruction Sheets, for the staff in the factory, in order to produce the work, which I had brought in each day. They sometimes made very expensive errors, due to the unclear instructions I had written.

140

My partner became so incensed by this needless waste of money and time that, one day; he stormed into my office, and forbade me to ever write out any more instructions, ever again. Although I was very annoyed at his temper outburst, and the disrespectful way he spoke to me, I soon realized that what he had said was the truth. I was writing badly, although I hadn't really noticed it. I was quite pleased at being relieved of this task, but I was also perturbed by the cause of this problem.

As an aside, my partner's name is Eric Sulter, and mine is Pepper, and many of our customers and friends, found this to be quite amusing. He and I are still very good friends, although we now live five hundred kilometers (three hundred miles) apart, and still laugh about the writing problem. He suggested to me, at the time, that I write in block letters whenever I have to make any notes on the job, so that there could be no confusion afterwards. I did this, and got into the habit of doing so, whenever I wrote anything down, after that.

I took his criticism to heart, and then set about writing everything in capital letters, from that moment onwards. I am quite good at it now, not taking that much longer than anyone else, to write things out. I only go wrong, when I get too anxious, and then I write unrecognizable rubbish.

Prior to the diagnosis, I became aware at each month-end, when signing my name on a pile of checks, that I was unable to sign more than about ten times, consecutively, before the signature got so bad I could not recognize it myself. At this point, the pen would not move any further, no matter how hard I tried to will it to do so. This may have been the same as the leg 'freezing', which I mention later. The problem appeared to be, that my brain could not control the hand movements. The illegibility did not occur, when I wrote in block letters, although, even this, tended to get smaller and slower as I wrote.

Insomnia

Whether my sleeping habit is work, or Pd related, I do not know for certain, but it is very common in Pd. As I have already stated, I developed the terrible habit of sleeping less than four hours a night, way back in the mid-seventies, when I first became aware of the depression problems.

Getting to sleep was not normally a problem, although, I did go through periods, where even that was difficult. I am sure that everybody experiences a problem falling asleep, *sometimes*. There were times, when I got up in the morning, convinced that I had not slept at all, during the night. At such times, my mind was invariably very active, after a busy day, spent wracking my brain for solutions to particularly difficult and challenging programming problems, or thinking about solving a dispute in the factory.

As a matter of interest, there were several occasions, when I dreamt of finding an error in one of the lines, deep inside a program, only to find the following day, that there really was such an error. When you consider that there were hundreds of thousands of lines of program, then this was quite incredible.

Getting a full night's sleep, became a rare occurrence, and seemed impossible to achieve any more. My most problematic time was three o'clock in the morning. I developed this habit of waking at or about that time, even after going to sleep as late as one o'clock. When I awoke, I usually became restless, starting to fidget, scratching my head and yawning. My mind soon became very active, and further sleep was impossible.

My doctor had, long ago, put me onto non-addictive sleeping pills, which I took for quite a while, against my better judgment. After having voluntarily ceased taking them, I was forced, on occasion, through sheer desperation, to have one, as I would have done anything for a full night's sleep. Unfortunately, even the sleeping pills, became useless, when I took them for more than three nights in a row. It became quite apparent to me, that the pressure of work had a major influence on my bad sleeping habit. When the pressure was high, I slept badly, if at all, but when it was down to acceptable levels, I was at least able to get my three to four hours a night. On each occasion, when I was reduced to taking the sleeping pills, I would sleep for eight or more hours on the first night, but by the fourth night, I was back to waking at three o'clock. On each occasion, I stopped taking the pills, at that point, as they did not help me to sleep. That was preferable to taking more and more pills at a time.

This sleeping pattern has continued to this very day. Although now since 2005, I sleep for an average of five to six hours a night, and even eight-hours occasionally. I take Trepiline tablets, every night now, which are non-habit-forming.

Intermittent Memory Loss

One day, someone will write a book of jokes about old age, and memory loss. When it happens to you, it isn't really funny, but neither is sexual dysfunction, about which we have all had a laugh or two. I am sure that medical practitioners are not sure themselves, whether memory loss is definitely Pd related or not. I have asked younger sufferers, if they have this problem, and have been told that they do. This does not prove the point, one way or the other. It is probably one of the most disconcerting problems, because it also helps to take away our dignity. It makes us appear to be fools, in front of our peers and family alike. Feeling foolish and inadequate, in front of anybody, encourages us to cease making contact with them, and that is the worst action we could possibly take. We need to keep up our contact with others. I do not want to generalize here, but when old or infirm people withdraw from society, their condition invariably deteriorates very quickly. It is therefore, not to be recommended.

This feeling of inadequacy came to the fore in 1996 or 97, when I started attending my first few support group meetings. People wondered which one of us had the Pd and as can be expected, they were generally rather skeptical of my claim to being a PwP. For the first couple of years of going to the Annual General Meetings of the Association, I was not able to accept the invitation to stand on the committee. This was because the very thought of speaking in public, and perhaps running meetings, was very intimidating indeed. The four company board meetings I attended every year were bad enough, but at least, in those meetings, I knew the company inside and out, and everybody in it. I was among my peers and they knew the problems I was having. However, working with strangers in a new environment, with people dealing with a disease, about which I knew very little, is a different kettle of fish altogether. So much has changed since then.

Since joining this association, I have had several embarrassing moments, due to memory loss. Not turning up to meetings, and forgetting to carry out promises, made at those meetings, were just a few of the more serious instances. Forgetting names and faces are still problems I face on a daily basis, and when working with voluntary workers, the least you can do is remember who they are. They are not the people I want to upset, but what can I do?

143

Another problem, relating to memory loss, is that the inability to remember important things, makes younger people impatient with us, and young people do not need too many excuses for getting impatient with older people. As I have already said, I have been very lucky with my children and grandchildren, as I still have a lot of contact with them, but even *they* get impatient with me, when I can't complete a sentence, or explain myself clearly.

On the lighter side; there have been three occasions in my life, since the mid-sixties, when I have been unable to remember Shirley's name, when trying to introduce her to strangers, whose names I also had already forgotten. This did not do my relations with Shirley much good, but as always, she forgave me, and we were able to laugh about it afterwards.

Involuntary Movements (Dyskinesia)

My feet constantly move, while lying in bed, or sitting in a reclining chair. I have heard this called 'restless legs' but don't know whether it is that or Dyskinesia. The movement is mostly circular in motion, with the added variations of up and down, and from side to side, rather like conducting an orchestra, with my feet. My feet hang over the end of my bed, because of my height, and when lying on my back, normally reading, the movement was, and occasionally, still is, almost constant. I noticed that music has a definite effect on this leg movement, as I seem to keep time with whatever is being played. If there is no music, the rhythm is in my mind.

Involuntary movements are not always limited to my feet. Although I was unaware of it at the time, my arms occasionally jerked involuntarily, while I was driving, sitting at the table, or eating. The jerking was not influenced by any outside stimulus, such as music. I was unaware of this fact until Shirley brought it to my attention, when consulting the neurologist. It was not a rhythmic movement, but a 'tic'.

I believe that this condition is not limited to Pd.

Irritability

This is not necessarily a true symptom of Pd either, but possibly, a behavioral problem, resulting from other symptoms. It could possibly be a sign of a personality change, which has taken place since diagnosis. It could also be part of the mood swing problem. I was always a very calm type of person. I was not ever subject to sudden mood changes or to fits of sulking. I seldom lost my temper, and I always tended to take the easy path in confrontational situations.

The reason why I put it in here is that I have been told that it could possibly be a result of hormone problems, which could very well be related to the Pd.

My irritability happens very suddenly, and often without any apparent reason. Sometimes the cause is obvious, but the reaction is not normal for me. Sometimes, when I try to fathom why I got irritable, I begrudgingly have to accept that something has happened, which did not suit me. In the past, such situations would not have caused a mood change, but now it does.

Shirley has been the person most affected by this symptom, and she has a fair idea of my true personality, after fifty years of marriage (2010). She is adamant that I was never like this before the Pd.

Upon reflection, this problem could be related to my frustration at not being able to do the activities, I used to be able to do. This may be so, but it seems to be too convenient. It is logical, because I really do get frustrated when I can't manage to loosen a button or tie my shoelace. But that frustration does not normally make me irritable. My irritability mostly seems to happen as a result of my interaction with other people. Because I spend most of my time with Shirley, it is not surprising that I often get irritable with her, but that is definitely not the case. I worship the ground she walks on. It is the situation, rather than the person, which is material in this analysis. Shirley sometimes asks if she is getting on my nerves, which is not even a remote possibility. As I said, it does not appear to be the person involved, who brings about the irritability, and that is always the situation.

Impatience should be my second name. On most occasions, I get impatient with myself, especially when I seem unable to explain simple things to others. When I make models, or paint intricate pictures, I have all the patience in the world.

Itchy Head and Torso

This symptom has bothered me for longer than I can remember. When I feel fatigued, I get a peculiar itching sensation, particularly on my head and face. This is not limited to my head, but less frequently happens on my upper torso as well. I become very agitated when it happens, in the movies and the theatre, where it causes those around me to become disturbed and distracted.

The itch is not a skin irritation, but a nervous irritation, which cannot be relieved by scratching, even though I can get to the very point, which appears to be itching.

I have asked others about this problem and not too many of them seem to be afflicted by it. I don't even know if this is a Pd problem, but because it is related to the nervous system, I have assumed that it is.

Lack of Awareness

I have become unaware of temperature changes. It can become warmer or colder, but I am not aware of it. I often get up during a winter night and work on my computer, still wearing my short summer pajamas. When Shirley gets up, she invariably asks if I am not cold which, in fact I am, but I am not aware of it. I find that my hands and feet are Ice cold to the touch, but I am not aware of it. I sleep the whole year round under a sheet, without a blanket. When it is really cold, I sometimes wake up, aware that I am shivering, but am not aware of it being cold. I put a blanket on, before going back to sleep, and often throw it off again, during the night, while Shirley has three blankets on. In the summer, when the room temperature becomes quite high; as long as I am not doing anything strenuous, I am not aware of the heat. Only when Shirley tells me it is very warm, do I realize that it is. I am aware, when I walk into a warm room, out of the cold, that it is warm, the same with the cold. I hate getting into a cold shower.

I do not often get the normal urge to defecate, and have to consciously try to get my stomach to work, but not always successfully. Sometimes, but quite rarely, I do get the urge to defecate; but that is invariably caused by some stomach upset.

This must all have something to do with the autonomic nervous system.

Lack of Facial Muscle Control

One of the symptoms, of which I was not aware at the time of diagnosis, was that I seemed unable to smile. This phenomenon manifested itself in my inability to show any emotion or exhibit any other facial expression.

When Shirley and I were at the neurologist together, on one of our visits, he mentioned this problem, and Shirley at once said that she had noticed it on me, although I was totally unaware of it.

I recently found a photograph, which was taken on the day that the Health and Racquet Club changed their security system, to credit card size membership cards, in 1993. The look on my face that day, four months after I was diagnosed, tells the whole story. The smile was only on one side of my face, and was nothing more than a grimace

Lack of Muscle Co-ordination

Back in the middle sixties, we used to take orphans out for a picnic in the countryside, together with fellow Round Tablers. We used to have a Barbeque (what we call a braai) for everybody, and we played football or cricket with the children. I became aware, when playing cricket, that I could not throw the ball directly to anyone. It went all over the place. I didn't follow this up with any doctor, but put it down to lack of practice.

During the seventies, I became aware of the fact that I was unable to throw a dart properly. I don't want to make light of any of the subject matter, but sometimes a little humor serves to lighten the mood. My brother says that I have *never* been able to throw a dart properly. Like many siblings, we are very competitive, and tend to be critical of one-another, although there is nothing we would not do for each other.

Sport does not really interest me. However, there are many 'games', as I call them, which play a vital role in community and family life, and whether you are good at sport or not, you can derive a lot of pleasure out of joining in. When I was younger, I used to be able to play darts quite well. At least, *I* thought I did. I wasn't ever a champion, or even a regular winner. In fact, I never won many games. However, regardless of how good or bad I was, I was not obviously physically challenged, and I enjoyed playing the game.

During the seventies, when I was already heavily involved in my new printing business, my family and I often visited one of Shirley's relations, in a nearby town. There, we invariably gravitated towards the dartboard, after a hearty meal, to play a friendly game or two.

Right from the outset, it was quite apparent to me, that something was very wrong with my dart-throwing capability. "You couldn't hit a cow in the ass with a shovel!" or words to that effect, were a common criticism. All of a sudden, my co-ordination had gone right out of the window. It wasn't that my aim was less reliable; I was simply not able to let go of the dart properly. The result was that the dart went anywhere *but* where I thought I was aiming, and more often than not, it missed the board completely. It did not do the walls or floors any good but, because it was so ridiculous, it became part of the fun. Still to this day, I cannot throw darts. I play darts every week, here at The Lodge, where we live. On most occasions, I get the booby prize for the lowest score. On one occasion, I actually won. This only goes to show that it is pure luck, whatever my score is.

At first, we all thought this was a huge joke and, seeing that I was a few years older than the rest of them, the playful remarks usually poked fun at old age and senility. I was not really put off by the ribbing I received; otherwise I would have avoided playing the game altogether. I did not seek medical advice at the time, because I didn't really give it any serious thought. I did not know that I had a neurological problem.

A little later in my life, this problem raised its ugly head again, but this time in a slightly different form. I experienced difficulty in throwing a ball up into the air, when serving in a game of tennis. The problem again was, that I could not let go of the ball properly.

That was not the only problem to raise its ugly head that day. The difficulty in serving the ball was exacerbated by a debilitating pain in my right shoulder, whenever I hit the ball with the racquet. A neurosurgeon later told me, while consulting him about this painful shoulder, that this was caused by osteoarthritis. However, many years later, another neurologist said that it is common to have stiff shoulders and pains in the joints with Pd.

At a later stage still, in 1981, I found that, playing lawn bowls was impossible for me, as well. I could not deliver the ball properly. This happened, when I was asked to join my fellow Rotarians in a game of Bowls, which I had never played before, other than the indoor version, on a carpet. I found that I had a similar problem to the dart throwing. The bowl would leave my hand and fly up into the air, landing with a resounding thump, on the green, causing an unwanted dent in the surface. That was not what serious bowlers regard as desirable behavior! Everybody assumed that I was playing the fool, and looked at me with disapproval. Even my family GP was there and didn't comment. When I told them that I was unable to let go at the appropriate time, they found it difficult to understand. So, after two more attempts to deliver the ball properly, I agreed to watch *them* play and refrain from damaging the greens any further.

Fortunately, I have other outlets for my enthusiasm, preferring music and art, to ball sports!

Legs Freezing

During the late seventies, when I was regularly attending my son's rugby matches at his school, I was astounded to realize that, after standing in one position, for a period of time, I was unable to move my legs. I was rooted to the spot, like a tree. It took a while before I was able to persuade my legs to move at all, but even then, only in a very restricted manner. When I *was* able to move, it was like walking in treacle. I could not get going properly, until the effects of the freezing wore off. I was mentally forcing my legs to move.

At the time, because of my back problems, and because I was under so much pressure, I did not give it a lot of thought. I didn't even tell my doctor about it, but the condition continued to haunt me for many years. I put it down to the fact that I had had that disc removed from my lower back, and since that time, standing still had always been uncomfortable, and even painful. I was also used to having nerves being pinched, in my back. When that happened, not only did I experience a lot of back and leg pain, I often experienced pains elsewhere, which I was told was "referred pain" from somewhere in the back. So, I avoided standing still, as much as possible, preferring to sit, with the result that the freezing did not happen too often.

Mood Swings

This symptom has only manifested itself over the past few years. I find myself becoming very short tempered with Shirley, of all people, for no rhyme or reason. I become very irritable and snap at her. It also happens with others, but not as often. In all fairness, the cause is always so petty that no person would say I was justified in getting bad tempered, over such a petty matter. I referred to irritability earlier on, but mood swings are more serious than temporary impatience.

I started taking Reminyl for this problem in 2006, which immediately solved it. Reminyl is normally prescribed for Alzheimer's disease, but there are many shared symptoms between these two conditions

Profuse Perspiring

When I have the opportunity, I like to potter around the house, and do all sorts of odd jobs, which seem to pile up imperceptibly, when my back is turned. I have been aware for many years that, when I am engaged in these activities, I perspire profusely, even when the temperatures are fairly low and the activity is in no way strenuous. My body acts as if I am in a state of extreme nervousness.

Also, when packing the car, before going away, or getting tickets at a railway station, I seem to become flustered, and perspire in this manner. I need to shower after each perspiring occurrence. I am wet from top to toe.

Respiratory Tract Infections

My family first went skiing in Austria, at the end of December 1979. I was then forty-five years of age, and had been having the muscle co-ordination problems, and the leg freezing problem, for quite a while. I came back from that holiday, and every subsequent skiing holiday, with a respiratory tract infection. The probable cause of this problem is my inability to keep the respiratory tract clear of mucus. Without sounding like a doctor, I believe the problem has something to do with the process, similar to 'peristalsis', whereby the body keeps the lungs and bronchial tract clear of mucus. This process does not necessarily work with Pd patients. The cold air and possibly some germs, while entering the lungs, cause an infection. Each year this infection appears to get worse. At least, as the patient, it appears to become more difficult to cure, and more difficult to carry on my normal activities. One of the occurrences took five courses of antibiotics, to get under control.

I have managed to bring down the incidence of bronchial infections by consciously clearing my air passages, as often as possible. This does not sound very nice, but I have no options.

I do not cough, or at least, try not to cough; I simply open my throat and push the air out of my lungs as fast as possible. This sounds much better, and it also avoids causing irritation of the larynx and throat.

I am led to believe that this is one of the major causes of death towards the end of Pd. I am not saying, or thinking, that this is the case with me, but I have to be very careful.

Restless Legs at Night

While lying reading in bed, my legs used to continually move around, as if searching for something. Sometimes it felt as if I were trying to pedal a bicycle or climb stairs. This movement tended to make me feel anxious and unsettled. It also annoyed Shirley, sometimes more than it did me.

This did not appear to be the same as the other foot movements. Dyskinesia does not cause any anxiety or discomfort. It is more annoying to others than to the patient.

Rigidity

At the outset, I have to admit that I do not understand this rigidity problem. It varies from day to day, not only in location, but also in nature. My body normally becomes fairly rigid in bed at night, as if rigor mortis has set in. I don't seem to move from the time I go to sleep, until the time I wake up in the morning. This may have something to do with the fact that, since my early youth, I have always gone to sleep in the same position in which I have woken up. Although; in my younger days, I always slept on my stomach. Now, I sleep on my left side, because of a blocked nose, and don't move all night.

After getting out of bed, it takes me a while to bend my legs and back sufficiently to enable me to dress myself. The same phenomenon occurs, after sitting down in a low easy chair, even for a short while. When getting up from the sitting position, it sometimes takes me quite a while to straighten, both my legs, and particularly my back, until I am in an upright position. Only then can I move properly. The joints appear to be at fault, although the muscles also seem to become rigid. I get the distinct feeling that old age has suddenly crept on!

Sometimes, while sitting in a chair, the phone rings, and I make a dash to pick it up, before the answering machine takes the call. I don't mind the machine taking the calls, but it is such a hassle, waiting for the answering message to finish, during which time, most of my callers seem to hang-up on me. In order to beat the answering machine, I get up and, without straightening up, walk as fast as I can, in a crouching position, to the phone. This is very uncomfortable, and a little painful.

Walking, has a peculiar effect on my body. When I set off on my bi-daily walk, it takes me some time to get my arms and legs moving satisfactorily; but while this is happening, the rest of my body seems to become totally rigid. When I finish my walk, the task of physically selecting the correct key for the door and putting it into the lock, seems almost impossible. The sensation in my hands is that same frozen feeling, which I have mentioned so often, even though my hands are as warm as toast. I next unlock the door, which is equally as difficult.

After I have wiped the sweat off my head and face, I set about some stretching exercises. One of these exercises involves grabbing hold of, first my one foot and then the other, while stretching my thigh muscles. This should be fairly easy, considering that I have just walked eight kilometers, but in practice, it is almost impossible. I first have to slowly bend my back, until my hands can touch my knees. Then I have to pull my knee up with one hand, until I can grab hold of my ankle with the other, which takes an age.

Once I get all my limbs moving on the walk, I am not conscious of the rigidity in the rest of my body.

This rigidity, as I have said, is something I do not really understand. For instance, when I have loosened up enough to be able to touch my toes (with bent knees), I would expect to be able to do so again after the next exercise, but this is not always possible. On many occasions, I have to go through the same loosening-up process again, before being able to touch my toes. When I say, 'Touch my toes', I mean with my knees and back bent to the limit.

Whether the joints and the muscles go rigid, or whether one or the other does, I do not know. As I have said, the rigidity is something about which I know very little. Today, I might be relatively mobile, but tomorrow the situation could be just the opposite. There seems to be no pattern to it, and I have never been able to trace a possible cause for it, other than the Pd.

The legs and the back are not the only culprits in this rigidity problem. Touching anywhere on my back is a time-consuming business, and not always guaranteed to work. If I want to touch the top of my spine, I have to use the other arm to help pull the elbow of that arm, over towards my head, thereby getting the hand, closer to the spine.

It is interesting to note that, even after sixteen years of walking, I still get noticeable stiffness in my muscles, the next day, as though I have done the walk for the first time in ages. This could have something to do with the rigidity, but having never discussed it with anyone, I am not in a position to make that statement.

Social Withdrawal

Shirley became aware of this phenomenon, which often occurred while I was relaxing with her in the evenings, even when we were with the family. When it happened, she used to ask me if something were wrong, or was something troubling me. I had the feeling that she thought I knew something, which I was keeping to myself, and she tried hard to drag it out of me. It even occurred a few times, while we were entertaining friends. On all of those occasions, I seemed to completely withdraw into a world of my own, a world, where nobody could reach me. Shirley used to tell me that I looked as if I were in a trance. This is more commonly associated with Alzheimer's disease, which hopefully, I don't have.

I was never aware of the problem myself. Whenever Shirley brought this remoteness to my attention, I was convinced that I had been listening to everything that was going on but, as I had nothing worthwhile to contribute to the conversation, I was content, just to be a listener. She, on the other hand, said that she used to watch me carefully, when I was in this state, and was convinced that I was not with her at all.

With the benefit of hindsight, I would not be at all surprised if this withdrawal was not simply due to plain exhaustion. After all, I was not in the habit of getting enough sleep, by normal standards, and I was working incredible hours. This state of withdrawal is very similar to what happens to us all, when we are about to go to sleep. The only reason why this does not quite match up to that situation is that when Shirley, or anybody else spoke directly to me, I did not react as if I had been awoken from a slumber. I reacted in the same way as anybody else would have done in a conversational situation.

It is very difficult for me to take part in a conversation, when there are more than two people involved. By the time I have thought of what I want to say, someone else has taken over and the conversation drifts away from what I wanted to talk about. Now, I stick my hand up in the air, and when people notice it, they stop and I say what I wanted to, whether it fits in with the subject matter at that point or not.

Speech Irregularities

During the eighties, the quality of my speech, changed. I had been quite adept at public speaking, often acting as master of ceremonies, at social functions. I was still entertaining the elderly people, in those days, telling jokes and being 'naughty'. However, when I got tired or stressed, my speech became slow, and rather labored and, at odd times, slurred. I had not really noticed this, but my family had. Knowing the strain under which I was working, they did not mention it to me. Only when the neurologist diagnosed Pd, and asked Shirley if she had noticed anything else, did she then inform him, and me, of the changes in my speech.

Frequently, my voice gradually gets fainter, during the course of the day; and by lunchtime, I can hardly speak above a loud whisper. At one stage, this became so pronounced, that I could no longer take phone calls, because the person on the other end, could not hear what I was saying. My voice soon returned however, after taking a rest, for at least an hour.

Speech articulation, at one stage, became problematic, when I was tired or stressed. I jumbled up my words, and even made utterances, which were not proper words at all. The result of this was that I started to feel like a real idiot, whenever I was called upon to address a gathering, at business meetings, or social functions. This was a further contributory factor to my loss of self-confidence. Although this does not happen very often now (2010), it does still occur.

What I have noticed is that, even when I can't talk louder than a loud whisper; I am still able to sing a strong note. This sounds to me like the difference in the control of the muscles, between when I sing and when I talk. The singing, I feel sure, is controlled by the conscious brain, while the talking is controlled by the subconscious. The volume is affected mainly by the volume of air passing through the larynx.

Losing my voice was a daily occurrence for me, at the time of writing the third edition of the book. At this time (2010), I have not been able to do my walking for the last fifteen months, because of leg injuries, further back problems, and recurring bouts of dizziness and vomiting, caused by the Meniere's syndrome. The voice and many other symptoms have returned to haunt me again, they will disappear, when I start to exercise again.

Tremors

As a child, I had a pronounced hand tremor. My parents put this down to the air raids over London, where we lived, and the constant bombing we endured, when I was small, which had a very traumatic effect on me at the time.

During the late eighties, these tremors became much worse. The tremors got to the stage, when locating and depressing the correct key on the keyboard of my computer, became a very hit-and-miss affair. That did not make my life any easier. Wrong keystrokes entered, when writing programs were not always easy to spot, and the time taken to de-bug those programs afterwards, became very problematic.

When waking up in the morning, I am in the habit of stretching my legs, before doing anything else, and in those days, when I did this, my whole body shook quite violently.

My next action, after stretching, is usually to lean out of bed and turn on the bedside radio. In those days, due to the tremor, I found this simple task very difficult to perform, and I quite often managed to knock over the glass of water, by my bed, while trying to turn the radio on.

As I have said already, my family doctor had thought, at one stage, that my hand tremors could possibly have been caused by panic attacks, because they only happened when I was trying to perform intricate tasks (Fine Motor Actions), or when I was performing on stage. They also happened when I became stressed. This was ruled out!

The tremors I experienced, early in the morning, were proof, to me, that the tremors in my hands had nothing to do with possible panic attacks, as there was no possible reason for me to be under any stress, at that time of the morning. There was therefore, in my opinion, nothing to cause me to panic. I certainly did not dread getting up.

While traveling overseas, carrying suitcases, with or without the built-in wheels, was very problematic. First, the hand carrying the case would start to shake; then it became unable to maintain its hold on the handle, and let go; but as the case began falling away from my hand, I immediately held on again.

These quick actions, of letting go and holding on, only lasted a few seconds, before I had to put the case down. However, I could then not let go of the handle at all. My hand froze in the position of holding onto the handle. I then had to use my other hand to prize the 'frozen' hand open.

Shirley was quite prepared to do all the carrying, but that was not practical. I didn't think of myself as an invalid, and I am too independent to ask others for help. Shirley thought that I was too mean with our money, to get a porter, but outside of South Africa, porters don't exist, at least, when you most need them. No! It wasn't a case of not wanting to pay someone to carry my case, it was probably a case of male ego, although I consider myself as not having an ego problem.

At the time of the diagnosis, my right thumb had a constant 'tic', when not in use, as did my left eyelid. This was not any sort of problem, only an inconvenience. This 'tic' was not a tremor. Why the one should have been on the right side and the other on the left, does not make sense.

Uncontrollable Emotional Occurrences

In May of 1982, I was present, at the unveiling of our newest and largest factory, down at Atlantis, in the former Cape Province of South Africa. I asked my business partner to make the opening speech, and switch on the presses. When these enormous machines started to churn out their product, at the rate of three hundred meters a minute, I was unable to control my emotions, and sobbed my heart out, in front of all those people. This had never happened to me, in my entire life. This problem has stayed with me to this very day.

Being present, anywhere near me, in a movie house, can be quite embarrassing, for everybody, including me. My emotional outbursts are quite audible and absolutely uncontrollable. When reading, I don't appear to become as emotional as I do, when watching a movie, or at live theatre. Making a speech is just as disturbing. When I get to a poignant passage, I become all choked-up, and cease to be able to continue. I know that this is fairly common amongst some people, but it had never happened to me, in my entire life.

At my sixtieth birthday bash, where I invited my friends and family to join me in celebrating life, I managed to deliver my message of thanks and appreciation to everybody who had helped to make Shirley's, and my life together, so fantastic. I

156

was managing fine, until the very end, when all I had to do was thank Shirley and my children. Fortunately for me, I had typed the speech out in full, and my daughter stepped in and read the remaining messages, one of which was to herself, which she left out. That was a bit of an anticlimax, to a wonderful evening. This problem is very common to older people, especially when they speak about their loved-ones. So, this could be age related, and not a Pd symptom at all, although I don't really think so.

Singing ballads, which either have sad music, or lyrics, causes me quite an emotional problem. First of all, I get into the ballad and, suddenly, without any warning, my throat becomes constricted, my voice cracks, and I am unable to continue. Silly! And embarrassing!

Something unusual happened to me, after diagnosis. Shirley and I were at the airport with our grandchildren, Matthew and Kristin, waiting for their parents to return from a trip to the USA. As it happened, our national athletics team was also returning home from the Olympic Games, on the same plane. There were crowds of people to welcome their heroes, and we could not get close enough to the barriers to be seen by my daughter, when she came out of the exit. So, I sat my seven-year-old granddaughter on my shoulders, so that she could see her mommy, when she arrived. We were about three or four people away from the barrier, but by then, both of us could see the exit clearly. Suddenly, I received a sharp dig in my ribs. I turned around to find a man, with a camera, who told me that he was a press photographer, and he wanted to get to the front of the crowd. I asked him if he had a press card with him; he told me that it was none of my business, and tried to push me out of his way. Normally, I would have let him pass, but on this occasion, I became very incensed by his attitude. I forgot that I had this little child on my shoulders, and I became engaged in a minor fracas with him. This frightened the life out of both my granddaughter and Shirley, who told me in no uncertain terms to pull myself together.

Afterwards, I was absolutely incredulous at my behavior, and must say that this was the first time that I had actually faced up to another person, ready to exchange blows.

By nature, I am not a fighter, and I have always believed that nothing has ever been solved by a fight. A fight only ever creates one more problem. You can understand from this that my behavior was totally out of character, and was, to say the least, very disturbing. I was on Prozac, at the time, for the depression, and we put it down to the medication, and my doctor immediately took me off the drug.

It is interesting to note that I am not the only person with Pd, who has experienced this change in personality. I have come across others with the same experience, during my many visits to support groups and individuals.

Watering Eyes

I will probably get shot-down by the Medical Profession, but, I am convinced that the problem of watering eyes is Pd related.

It happens, mainly when I am tired, but not always. I am invariably in bed, or on a chair, reading; or else I am in the car, driving. The thought has occurred to me that the watering may be caused by my eyelids, which may not be blinking at the required rate, allowing the eyes to become dry and irritated, thus causing the watering. I have tried to overcome this by consciously blinking, but I find it difficult to do while I am reading.

It has been suggested that my eyes need testing, but I have had this done, many times, and there is nothing wrong there. This problem is invariably accompanied by fits of deep yawning.

Approximate Progression Timetable of My Pd

This book was first written, ten years after I was diagnosed, and nearly thirty years after the first symptoms appeared. it was very difficult to remember, when each symptom first started. I found that I was best able to relate them to where I was living, when each one appeared. Some of the dates are very accurate, because of an event, which took place then. Symptoms marked with an asterisk, still happen, but, other than choking, do not cause me any great problems.

Symptoms, which Started, while in our Kimberley home"

| Early 60's | *Unable to let go of a ball properly, while trying to throw it. (Muscle coordination) *Became regularly constipated. |
| 1968 | *Found that I was unable to write properly |

Symptoms, which Started, while in our Springs home:

| 1971/2 | *Unable to let go of a dart Properly. (Coordination) |

Mid 70's	Unable to move my feet, after standing still for a While. (Freezing) *Unable to walk over uneven surfaces. (Still Happens if I don't concentrate). *Diagnosed with depression. *Noticed that I constantly turn right, when I want to turn left. *Unable to clear trachea, resulting in infections.
1981 1982	*Unable to let go of the bowl properly, whilst playing lawn bowls. (Coordination) *Became very emotional, and actually cried, at the opening of new factory. Have been unable to control my emotions, even for unlikely causes, such as nice music and sad stories.
Mid 80's	Unable to manipulate my fingers. (Freezing) Hands froze in a fixed position, after carrying heavy objects, such as suitcases. *Found that I was unable to handle conflict situations. *Found multi-tasking very difficult *Started to regularly knock objects over, at the dining table. I started to become 'remote', not appearing to be with everybody, but away somewhere else. When questioned by my wife, I always said I was listening to everybody, but was unable to join in the conversation. *Get cramps in my feet, when getting into bed and before sleeping. *Started Supinating on my right side.

Symptoms, which Started, while in our Sandton home:

Late 80's	Tremors got so bad that I was unable to accurately depress the keys on the computer keyboard. I shook so badly I could not demonstrate my Computer system to a prospective client. Lost my balance, while wandering around the gym, and at home. When under pressure, I perspired very badly around Head and torso. Started falling asleep, at work. Became very fatigued, during the daytime. *Developed bad posture and a bad gait.

	*Became unable to access words, while talking *Found I could not remember names and dates Started to garble my words. Started dribbling on my pillow, at night. Started making involuntary arm movements. Started having 'restless legs' at night *Battled to put socks and shoes on. (Rigidity) *Had difficulty reaching my toes with both hands, even with my knees bent. (Rigidity) Battled to do up buttons. Battled to dress myself. Unable to smile properly. Struggled to concentrate at work. *Found swallowing certain food was difficult. Had to cover food with gravy or sauces. *Started to choke quite regularly, both during meals and when saliva ran into my windpipe. *My eyes started watering, mainly in bed at night, while reading. This is often accompanied by fits of yawning.
1992 Mid 90's	Diagnosed with Pd. *Noticed that my right heel was held off the ground all the time I sat at my desk. *When driving, my toes are clenched tight. Can rectify it, but goes straight back, when not thinking about it. *Lost my libido, and experienced erectile problems.

Symptoms, which Started, while in our Retirement Village:

Mid 2000	*I started experiencing mood swings, getting cross over silly little incidents, and threw my toys out of the cot. I was given Remenyl for this. *Started to take trepiline for the insomnia. *Started having more than the normal occurrences of biting my tongue and the insides of my mouth.

Appendix 2
Supporting Letters
Putting Your Mind to Improving Your Health

Good health is so difficult to define, but it is more than just the absence of disease. It reflects a state of mental, social and physical fitness and well-being, and is strongly influenced by one's lifestyle.

John is an extraordinary person! I soon learned this, watching him attempt his goal, to overcome Parkinson's disease to the best of his ability. By making an effort to overcome the neuro-degenerative disorder of Parkinson's, John has improved the quality of his life to the point where he no longer appears to require drug therapy.

John adopted a healthier lifestyle and, as the months went by, his condition gradually changed. By joining my branch of Run/Walk for Life, in 1994, it gave me immense gratification to witness how he overcame his disability. It was through his own self-help and total commitment to exercise that his fitness and health improved.

Initially, I could imagine the frustration John must have felt, being inflexible and unable to maintain his balance, like his fellow members, but this was his challenge in life - to put his mind to it, and become one of the top walkers, excelling in time trials and a walking race!

I frequently invited John to present talks at our inter-branch 'Get-together' breakfasts, in order to motivate others, who had no physical disabilities at all! These talks were enlightening to everyone and as he stood there talking each time, I felt a sense of pride and joy.

With the support of his wife, Shirley, his family and self-commitment to his cause, he did it! I have the greatest admiration for John. I have no doubt this book will help many people, who find themselves in similar circumstances, improve their own quality of life.

John, it was a privilege to have helped you in my small way and you can be proud of what you have achieved through your own mind-set.

Shirley Soll. Run/Walk for Life, Wendywood.

A Journey of Self-discovery and Conquest

I am privileged to call John my "FRIEND". John joined my Art Class, two years ago. A victim of Pd, he was very insecure about his ability to hold a drawing implement steady – his choice of medium was the pencil crayon, which was easier to hold; his format size was small, as was his lack of confidence in his ability to execute what he saw and intellectually interpreted. He was very aware of his "handicap".

The first art class John attended, was held at the Zoo. John battled with a shaky hand, preventing him from drawing any recognizable lines on paper. He became very stressed, not only with the hand tremor, but also with the reality that animals would not stand still. Somehow, he managed to find a method of drawing the animals in a way that left the observer with no doubt about the subjects.

John is enthusiastic, has a wonderful sense of humor and is able to laugh at himself. He is also stubborn and tenacious. This book celebrates John's journey from victim to victor! John rose to every challenge I posed, in my perceptually based art lessons. I expected him to give of his best and he excelled himself. He dismissed no problem as impossible to solve.

It has been such a pleasure watching John evolve into a confident Artist, where his ability to execute fine detail in both two and three dimensional artwork is impressive, - which is hardly surprising as the man himself is impressive, showing courage, determination and willpower, which has taken him far beyond the confines of his "handicap".

John has not only proved to himself, but to all of us, that with motivation, dedication, belief in himself and willpower, you can conquer your fears, limitations and handicaps. I believe that the greatest gift you can give students is to show them that you believe in them. Thank you John for proving that there is no limit to your ability to succeed, when you believe in yourself! It has been a privilege, as your teacher, to share your journey of self-discovery and conquest!

Estelle McIlrath – Art Teacher.

Letter from Jules Klette

6 September 2002

Dear Sheila

You asked about my reaction to John Pepper's talk (demonstration really) at our Parkinson's meeting in June?

While cursing my affliction roundly and often, I have to admit to being one of the better-off sufferers; due mostly to a care giver and a family who have not allowed me to capitulate. Also, I have been fortunate enough to have access to doctors, drugs, physiotherapist, and occupational therapists and vitamin supplements aplenty. All this, and yet, suddenly we have John Pepper in our midst, showing us how much more can be done on our own to get on top of this disorder. How to walk, how to talk, how to manipulate eating utensils? Most of us have read casually about these things, perhaps even tried out one or two of the 'control' suggestions; but what an inspiration it was to have the example of John right here with us. The impact was tremendous. Apart from being able to identify and work at several of my own needs I was able to witness the walking lessons given to Yvonne. She was made to heel toe, heel toe, lift her feet, swing her arms..............the results were extraordinary. In the short space of time of approximately twenty minutes she was transformed from a serious shuffler to a walker. She had found it exhausting but was resolved to keep it up.

So if anyone wants to know whether I thought John Pepper's visit was a success, the answer is a resounding **YES.**

Yours sincerely

Jules Klette

Letter from Wilna Jeffery
P.O.Box 650413, Benmore, 2010 South Africa.
09 May 2008

Dear John,

Your book inspired me so much that I joined 'Walk for Life' back in 2003, due to the emphasis you placed on the importance of exercise. I still do my Walk for Life, and I still play regular golf, although, at the time of first meeting you, I was going to give it up, because of the shocking way I was playing.

Your inspiration made me take a hard look at my lifestyle and I have not looked back since. I still take only three Stalevo pills per day, and am still able to play my golf, play regular bridge with my friends, and live a perfectly normal life.

So, after being face to face with you, on three separate occasions, my whole attitude towards Pd has changed into something very positive. My family and friends have all remarked on my improvement, since my first meeting with you. You have given me the courage to live a perfectly normal life, despite Parkinson's, and the confidence to face this condition head-on and not let it get the better of me.

You shared your experiences with me, and in doing so, I found that the tremor in the hand, the aching muscles and the dragging foot, which tripped over the smallest obstacles, were no reason to give up on life! I have searched very hard to see these symptoms in you, but have failed. You have fought and won the battle, and it has given me such hope to do the same.

You taught me two vital lessons. The first was how to walk properly, in order to prevent the dragging foot. The second was how to hold a glass with confidence, without spilling its contents, not that I am a great drinker. You are extremely approachable and natural, and I have felt very comfortable asking you many of my unanswered questions, to which you have given very knowledgeable, yet heartfelt answers, as you have truly experienced what I am going through.

Not only has my physical being improved tremendously, but my mind is that much more alert too. Thank you John Pepper!

Yours Sincerely,

Wilna Jeffery.

Letter from Grace Ravno

Dear John

I belong to the Durban Support Group in Westville. A while back, you came to our meeting and gave a very interesting talk to us. I was interested particularly in hearing you say that if one concentrates completely on one thing, you can actually do it without shaking. You gave a few examples like carrying a very full glass of water and not spilling it, etc.

I was diagnosed with Pd 6 years ago, and although I am not too shaky, I have been getting worse. So I tried the concentration thing, and was thrilled to be able to pick up and carry a full glass of water across a room! I'm also a pretty dab hand serving drinks, when I am on "Bar Duty" at our bowls club. Then I decided to try this in another way. We all know how small our handwriting gets, and also how illegible. Well, I have been doing Calligraphy for many years, but had virtually packed my pens and paper away because I saw no future there. Until one day I focused totally on my pen, the style I wrote it in, and I shut out all outside noises - and voila! My Calligraphy was as good as ever! I have been asked to do various writings in various styles and as long as I am completely focused and don't speak to anyone, I am coping very well again. The first project I did, once I got started, was for a dear friend who had forgotten I had Pd. Her expectations were very high, and because of her confidence in my ability, I found I had risen to the challenge with no problem!

So, thank you for encouraging us in overcoming our short-comings, and for giving us an extra prop to use to accomplish what we set out to do. If you ever meet me at a cocktail party and you see how full my wine glass is, I would suggest you don't come and talk to me, because once my focus is taken off the glass, you could be the recipient of a shower of wine!

I am enclosing herewith a copy of "Be thou my vision....." all long verses of it, which I did a few weeks ago. Thank you again for your help in finding a way to overcome "the shakes".

Grace Ravno

Letter from Bianca Turner

20 Skemer Street, Malmesbury, 7300.

11ᵗʰ August 2009

Dear Mr. Pepper

My father, Ian Fleming, at 81 years of age, is proof that a Parkinson's diagnosis can be reversed! I always say he's the 'wunderkind' of the support group.

Actually, he has taken ownership of his life and condition, and does what he is told. He exercises religiously, (walking for gross motor and specific hand/arm etc exercises) and always takes his Carbilev before meals.

He also has outside interests to stimulate himself - specifically he wants to publish a book he is working on regularly. Also, he plays bowls occasionally and reads to my children, his grandchildren, almost every evening for +- 20 minutes.

I always say, "Now we have a road-map" – the diagnosis is not a death sentence but a pointer to the journey forward.

Thank you for your fascinating, encouraging book, for coming today, for sharing the story of your life.

Every time one new person manages Parkinson's with skill and optimism, it's one new life given special direction.

Bless you for what you do; may every success accompany you.

Kindest regards

Bianca Turner. (nee Fleming)

Appendix 3
Exercise Is Not Optional, It Is Mandatory.
SPRING Times No 40. Page 14-16.

The World Parkinson Congress[10], the first of its kind, took place from February 22nd to 26th, 2006 at Washington Convention Centre, USA, attracting some 3,200 participants, 1,100 of whom were patients or caregivers.

The Congress supported by the Movement Disorder Society, the National Institute of Health, U.S. Army Medical Research Acquisition and over 100 professional and patient organizations from all over the world, was unique not only in size and scope but also in that it brought together patients, caregivers and many of the world's leading Parkinson's experts, doctors and scientists.

Michael Kelly, a SPRING member, who attended the Congress, has written this article for SPRING Times.

With almost 200 papers to choose from, it was not an easy task for me to select those that might be of special interest to patients. In taking the subject of exercise as being worthy of special attention, I have singled out three papers for comment based on the following criteria:

- Scientific importance of medical information
- Originality of content
- Immediate relevance for patients

The three papers are supplemented by an addendum, based on work currently in progress at the University of Frankfurt. Taken together, the material presented provides good grounds for a **major re-evaluation of the role of exercise in patient therapy.**

In the first talk entitled **How exercise affects the brain: Towards a rationale for exercise-induced protection,** Dr Michael Zigmond from the University of Pennsylvania spoke about the benefits of exercise, pointing out that it has been accepted for a long time that exercise is recommended for people suffering from numerous conditions, including cardiovascular problems and diabetes. He referred to the fact

---

[10]http://spring.parkinsons.org.uk/images/stories/SpringDigest/2006/40
_3_ExerciseIsNotOptional.pdf

that studies carried out showed that the incidence of Alzheimer's disease, stroke and PD **was lower for those who exercised regularly compared to control groups.**

The question is: **What is it about exercise that confers a benefit?** The work of Dr Greeno at the University of Illinois was referred to. He has been testing, a) animals walking fast or running, b) animals having to balance on a tightrope to obtain food, and c) couch potato animals relaxing all day. It has been found that **running** very significantly increases blood vessel density in the brain, with enhanced flows of blood improving the supply of nutrients and facilitating removal of waste. Furthermore, the tightrope group showed an increase in the number of synapses and overall, exercise increased the supply of survival or trophic factors. Running or fast walking had no effect on synapses and tightrope walking had no effect on blood supply. So, the type of exercise taken; needs to be considered, when designing a program. Reference was made to the work of Dr Carl Cotman at the University of California, showing that there is **an increase in survival factors in the brain with exercise.**

The question then becomes: **what kind of exercise is needed and how much?** The answer is: **"lots of different types of exercise".**

Dr Zigmond then went on to talk about an animal model using the 60HDA neurotoxin (6 hydroxy dopamine). In a series of elegantly designed experiments using rats (referred to by Dr Zigmond as animals with front-wheel-drive) with individual forelimbs immobilized in casts and thus with the rat being forced to use a particular limb, it could be shown that forced exercise prior to or immediately after lesioning, with 6OHDA and continued for 7 days, **could completely counteract the toxic effects of 6OHDA.** Video clips of this phenomenon were shown for various configurations and provided an impressive demonstration of the benefits of exercise. If exercise was initiated seven days after lesioning, no beneficial effects occurred. Dr Zigmond could give no precise data on how long the effects lasted and how intensive the exercise had to be. This aspect will be referred to later.

The second talk with the somewhat unwieldy title: **The effect of high-intensity exercise using body-weight supported treadmill training on neuroplasticity and functional recovery in individuals with Pd** was given by Dr

Beth Fisher from the University of Southern California. Dr Fisher has been involved for some years in translating over animal movement research for use in human applications. She spoke about the re-modeling that the brain is capable of, pointing out that, in recent years, a much greater degree of plasticity has been found to exist than was formerly thought to be the case. This applies not only to animal models but also to stroke and spinal injury models.

Dr Fisher reported on studies of mice using MPTP (a neurotoxin, causing immediate damage to dopaminergic neurons) in which one group receiving MPTP was exercised intensively for 30 days, a second group receiving MPTP did no exercise and a third group exercised without receiving MPTP. **It was found that the MPTP group, which was forced to exercise, caught up with the non-MPTP exercise group and, in terms of speed and endurance, could match them after 30 days. This provides powerful evidence of the benefits of exercise in an animal model.**

For exercise-testing of patients, use was made of a treadmill with an overhead bodyweight-support suspension harness to allow high-intensity exercise without any danger of falling or injury. Patients were divided into three groups: a high-intensity exercise group with MET 3.5 and above, a low-intensity group with MET below 3.0 and a no-exercise control group (1 MET=1kcal/kg, h). Testing was carried out in 24 sessions, each of 60 minutes duration, over a period of 8 weeks.

The outcomes of the exercise were measured in terms of changes in disease severity, functional performance (stair climbing, stand/sit movements) and brain function testing. This latter test, carried out using Trans-cranial Magnetic Stimulation (TMS) techniques, provided the most significant indications of the benefits of exercise. At various levels of stimulation, TMS was used to provide a Motor Evoked Potential (MEP) response, with peak-to-peak maximum amplitude and cortical-spinal rest time (Silent Period Duration, SPD) being measured independently in both brain hemispheres. This enabled a comparison to be made between the more the less affected sides in Pd patients and between Pd patients and healthy controls. SPD tends to be shortened and MEP shows higher peak-to-peak rest values (hyper excitability) in Pd.

Comparison between pre- and post-exercise readings showed that exercise led to a convergence to normal values

in Pd patients, with the higher intensity exercises having the greatest effect.

A third very engaging talk entitled **People with Pd should have weekly Parkinson exercise classes for the rest of their lives** was given by John Argue from San Francisco. John is a former actor and, for the past 23 years, a physical therapist, working with People with Pd.

His approach to exercise and movement is a very practical one, using the activities of everyday life to counteract the restrictions imposed by Parkinson's. A book he published in 2000 has sold over 20 000 copies and he now has a DVD out containing details of this program.

As an actor, John is able to slip into the role of a Person with Pd (PwP) and gave a completely convincing performance in terms of posture and movement. His somewhat unconventional approach to physical therapy involves three main headings: **Stretching** – as a preventive measure, countering foreshortening and restrictions of movement, **Strength** – to prevent muscle atrophication and to maintain ability to perform movement, along the lines of 'use it or lose it', **Movement strategy** – managing movement such that one is mindful of the sequence of actions required to complete the execution of a task. Examples shown included motion sequences associated with sitting down on a chair, rising from a supine position etc. Such sequences are executed automatically, when a person is healthy, but can pose severe problems for a PwP.

John's program involves 10 lessons, the first 5 of which are performed lying or sitting. Video clips with examples of straight stretch, rotational stretch, tilt side stretch etc. were shown.

Very early on in therapy, PwPs are given fall training, long before falls become a factor in disease progression. Patients are shown how to protect their face and head and how to mitigate the effects of falling.

John emphasized the importance of group therapy, not only in terms of the fellowship created among patients and benefits accruing from getting a sense of **control over the disease**, but also in as far as it gives caregivers time to rest and recuperate.

Addendum: As a spin-off from programs developed for performance improvement of top-class athletes, the University of Frankfurt has been carrying out extensive testing on the effects of various types of motion stimuli. One such program has been aimed at off-season training supplementation for downhill alpine skiers. This has led to development of the so-called Zeptor, a treadmill-like device with two oscillating footplates. This has been in use for past 2-3 years in specialized Parkinson clinics in Germany. Extensive tests in Germany and in Spain have shown it to have positive effects due to interactions between variable-intensity semi-stochastic (random) oscillations and neuro-muscle systems.

Dr Haas, a researcher in the Institute of Sport Medicine in Frankfurt University, has reported on tests showing that exercise/movement of a particular type can lead to nerve growth factors (NGF) being released by nerve cells (through activation of muscle sensors referred to as spindles). NGF initiates a cycle leading to enhanced formation of proteins, thereby assisting in **neuron survival and growth**. Increased physical activity is thus found to protect nerves but NGF release is dependent on the type and range of movement. Exercise carried out while standing have little or no effect on NGF, swimming has a small effect and treadmill exercises give good results. To achieve the best results, exercises should meet the following criteria:

- Be quasi-rhythmic but with a stochastic element (a degree of randomness)
- have a frequency of 1-10 Hz, about 5 Hz is optimal
- involve a learning situation (complexity) and, if possible,
- have an element of spatial variability.

Swimming is apparently too slow to be of major benefit but jogging/walking fast* (over uneven ground) would seem to come close to the ideal. Completely rhythmic or repetitive movements (such as might arise for example when holding a pneumatic tool) lead only to fatigue, with no beneficial effects on the nervous system. **To get maximum physiological and neurological benefit, it would appear to be important to exercise on a regular basis because muscular degeneration begins within some days of stopping exercise.**

The exercise sessions should involve a challenging degree of intensity, duration and complexity, factors that will vary widely depending on the abilities and impairment status of the individual.

Summary: While the benefit of exercise has been appreciated for many years, only in recent times has research begun to unravel the mechanisms underlying this phenomenon and to provide a differential evaluation of what different kinds of exercise can do. Findings that exercise can counteract the effects of neurotoxins and can lead to increases in nerve growth factors are especially encouraging. **By establishing a solid basis for the benefits of exercise, it is hoped that patients on a wider front will be encouraged to include it as an integral part of their daily routine**.

Articles supplied by Northwest Parkinson's Foundation Post:

To Exercise or Not: That is the Question!

By Peter B. Sparrow
Reproduced from The Wisconsin Parkinson's Association
Publication The NETWORK, Winter 2009-03-05

With a degree as a physical therapist assistant and greater than 20 years in practice, I was not a foreigner to the medical field, when I was diagnosed with Parkinson's disease (Pd). I had always been an active person. My life included enjoying cross-country skiing, tennis, whitewater canoeing, hiking, camping, rock climbing, bicycling, swimming, sailing and horseback riding. I also was active with gardening, landscaping and home maintenance. Being married to an occupational therapist, I tended to think about exercise as a side benefit of everyday activities as well as work.

Gradually, as I got older, my wife and I adopted two children and then I realized that my life was becoming changed by Pd. All activities that I had enjoyed as functional activities became more difficult and I had less time for them, because of family obligations. As the years passed, I gained weight, and because of over-use of the "non-" Pd leg, I ended up tearing the distal posterior tibialis tendon. The result of this tear was a decreased ability to walk and consequently an increase in body weight along with general de-conditioning (decreased strength, flexibility, endurance and flexed posture). My life changed on December 3, 2007 with surgery on my calf muscle and non-weight bearing postoperative.

My physical therapist, who specializes in Pd, convinced me to try an exercise program at the Waukesha YMCA. Reluctantly, I went to the program and started to do exercises that I had done, during my professional career, previously prescribed for my own clients, who had Pd. Why did I have to pay for someone to watch me do exercises that I already knew? Besides, they were not functional activities. I found that I am consistent with the class, because I pay for it. My cardiovascular endurance, range of motion and strength have all improved and I lost 10 pounds. The class acts as a support group and the volunteers who run the program are neat professionals and students.

The class is a nice social break and I recommend that people with Pd try a class near them. If there is not one in your area, find a physical therapist, who will lead an exercise program in a facility that has treadmills available. The *Wisconsin Parkinson's Association* will advise you and the therapist on how to get a class started. The squeaky wheel gets the grease, so keep asking.

In addition, get interested in life. Pretend that you are training for the Olympics. Have mental activities like board games, cards, pictorial and word puzzles. Have physical activities, have social activities. Volunteer.

You will fatigue, but you can get beyond that. People with a neurological insult will feel this way. After all, your body has to work harder than the "normal person" to get the same result.

I progressed to full weight-bearing work out on the treadmill for half an hour (backwards, sideways and forwards), and do floor/chair/ stand/ walk exercises. I used to use a rolling walker all the time. Now I only use it occasionally in the evening, when I feel my posture failing and/or I have a long or uneven terrain to navigate. It is handy to sit on at a soccer game or at dances and plays. My children are twelve and fifteen years old, while I am a mere 61. **I now ride a bicycle, walk on uneven terrain, without any device, climb stairs with or without a rail, lay tiles, drive a car or lawnmower, canoe, sail, bowl, use a chain-saw, do light carpentry and masonry, swim, coordinate building projects and play chess.** You have to be careful with your activities, so clear it with your professional (neurologist, physical therapist, occupational therapist, athletic trainer and chiropractor) before starting any new physical activity.

After a long day of activity, I am wiped! I plop myself down in my recliner, that goes perfectly flat and I enjoy a rough foot massage by my faithful dog with her sand paper tongue.

What can you do with your extra time?

Potential for exercise to slow Parkinson's progression

23 October 2009

New results, presented at the Society for Neuroscience's annual meeting in Chicago this week point towards the profound effects that exercise may have on the brain. In studies conducted by researchers at the University of Pittsburgh in the US, exercise is able to protect the brains of monkeys against chemicals that researchers usually use to mimic Parkinson's.

Testing exercise for Parkinson's

Over a period of 3 months, monkeys were divided into groups that either ran, jogged or sat on a treadmill for an hour every day, 5 days a week. After this training period, all the monkeys were given MPTP, a chemical which attacks the nerve cells that are lost in Parkinson's. These nerve cells produce dopamine, a chemical messenger that helps regulate movements. The MPTP successfully killed dopamine producing nerve cells in the monkeys that sat still. They developed a slowness of movement that is typical of Parkinson's. But in the brains of monkeys that had been running, MPTP had almost no effect. Their dopamine-producing nerve cells survived and the monkeys were protected from the Parkinson's symptoms, that normally occur. Even after another 6 weeks, brain scans showed that exercising animals had virtually normal levels of dopamine in their brains.

What does this mean?

Dr Kieran Breen, Director of Research and Development at the Parkinson's Disease Society, comments: "These new studies provide tantalising glimpses of the potential exercise has to slow the progression of Parkinson's – something no current treatment can." Now, further studies are crucial to understand exactly how exercise affects the brain, and how we can harness the power of exercise, to develop better treatments and therapies for people with Parkinson's."

Exercise is Medicine for the Parkinson's Brain

BY Patrick J. Hogan, D.O.

Despite the tremendous capacity of medications to improve function and quality of life in Pd, their benefits have limits. That's why, in addition to medications, a comprehensive approach to treatment necessarily includes **good nutrition, stress control and especially** *an exercise program.*

Exercise has long been considered a means to condition the muscles and heart. However, we now know **exercise in Pd also has direct benefit on the brain.**

Documented structural and chemical changes occur in the brain, with exercise, resulting in improvements in function beyond what is derived from medication alone.

The list of benefits is impressive. Exercise contributes to:

- **Improved postural stability with a resultant decreased rate of falls (and less injury if falls do occur)**
- **Improved bone strength**
- **Improved standing ability and gait motion**
- **Improved fine-motor dexterity**
- **Improved stamina and reduced daytime fatigue**
- **Improved sleep quality**
- **Improved control of mood and stress**
- **Improved cognitive function of memory and attention**
- **Improved bowel, urinary and sexual function**
- **Improved appetite and prevention of excessive weight loss**
- **Improved weight control for those with excessive weight**
- **Improved cardiovascular health and endurance**
- **Improved perception of quality of life**

Studies show that a challenging exercise program **increases the number of brain cells as well as the connections between brain cells – with resulting improvement to the symptoms of Pd, and slowing in the Pd progression.**

In studies, for which animals with induced Pd were divided into two groups, one that exercised and one that didn't, the exercising animals exhibited a **reversal** of the Parkinson's pathology, whereas Parkinson's steadily progressed in those that did not exercise.

We have long recognized the benefits of exercise for Pd, in clinical practice; this thinking is now backed by scientific evidence that **exercise produces chemical and structural changes in the brain that enhance how the brain functions.**

Studies also show that exercise improves brain function in those with memory impairment either from normal aging or from dementias, due to Alzheimer's or Pd.

It has been shown that those in a regular exercise program **have 40% less memory impairment** over the long term than those who don't exercise regularly.

Current research is investigating what types and quantities of exercise produce the most positive effects in the brain. The research suggests that it may not take very much exercise, but that the **exercise needs to be consistent and challenging, rather than casual and unvaried**, for the best brain results.

This is because, when challenged, the brain responds with changes to make it easier next time the challenge occurs. This is a slow and steady process but amazingly effective over time.

Exercise Guidelines for Parkinson's Patients

Waiting to exercise each day until you "get to it" is the best way of *never getting to it*. Consider exercise as important as your medications and schedule time for it every day.

Exercise with enough frequency and intensity – not to mention variety – to challenge the brain into responding by producing the chemical changes needed to generate new cells and synapses.

Keep in mind that exercise requiring a coordinated effort provides the greatest challenge to the brain.

Depending on your capabilities, you might consider some or all of the following: treadmill walking or running, tai chi, dancing, biking (stationary or otherwise), water aerobics, and guided physical therapy exercise.

Dance has proved particularly helpful in stimulating both the cognitive and physical capacities of the brain.

It's helpful to have a local Pd exercise group that meets weekly to supplement your daily exercise program.

Therapists at St. Joseph's Hospital in Tacoma maintain a weekly exercise program for the local Pd community that has been very successful, over the past few years. (More information about this program is available by calling 253-426-4400.)

You may find there is a similar or comparable exercise program in your own community.

At its optimal level, treatment Of Pd is a team approach between care provider and patient.

Near-daily physical exercise, is among the very best ways people with Pd can contribute to their own care and improve their long-term quality of life.

Appendix 4
More Information on MAO-B Inhibitors

SPRING Times No. 41, October 2006 Page 15:

Synapses – Collecting Thoughts
By John Telford

Synapses connect nerve cells – so, in a sense, they connect thoughts. In this edition of ST, as in many others, articles written quite separately have born an unexpected relationship with each other. A discussion in one has serendipitously thrown light on another. The thoughts crossing the synapses in this edition relate to oxidative stress, neuroprotection and monoamine oxidase inhibitors such as selegiline

The article by Michael Kelly on exercise in the last edition prompted John Pepper to write in about how he believes regular, strenuous exercise has helped keep his Pd symptoms at bay. He happened to mention in correspondence that he had used selegiline (Eldepryl) as a monotherapy for many years (i.e. without any levodopa). I was not aware that there was any advantage in using selegiline on its own but another of our regular contributors had also used it in this way. But there should be no surprise about this mode of use. Monoamine oxidase type B inhibitors (MAO-B inhibitors) certainly **slow down the degradation of the dopamine in the brain** that has resulted from levodopa administered, as Pd therapy. But it will of course also extend the life of the dopamine produced naturally by the neurons. Therefore: **in the early stages of the disease, when dopamine production has started to decline, an MAO-B inhibitor can help to conserve what dopamine is still being produced by the cells, not yet affected."**

The link between ideas relates to Flora Hill's article above[11] on alpha synuclein. In the model 2 that she describes, free dopamine is seen as harmful. Not in itself but because of the highly reactive oxygen species which are formed when excess of it is metabolized. The first stage of a major route in the metabolization of dopamine is the action of a monoamine oxidase – the very enzyme that compounds like selegiline act against. (The relatively new drug, rasagiline, which is marketed

---

[11] *Flora Hill wrote an article DeNDRoN (Dementias and Neurological Diseases Research Network)*

as Azilect is of the same class.) Model 2, then, suggests that such drugs may help with neuroprotection, by inhibiting the harmful degradation of any dopamine, that has escaped being re-absorbed.

So the question is; has selegeline contributed to the slowness of PD progression that John Pepper has experienced? Well, we have to be cautious. One swallow does not make a summer, and conclusions cannot reliably be drawn from anecdotal evidence. After all, there still remains some question of whether John Pepper really has 'standard' Pd. Instead, the correct answer is what Flora proposes: that further research is done, firstly, to confirm the results of the trial she quotes, which point to MAO-B inhibitors being neuroprotective and second, to determine whether they are neuroprotective by the mechanism she outlines.

The following information was supplied by the *Parkinson's Post, Published by the Northwest Parkinson's Foundation*[12]:

On May 16, 2006, the Food and Drug Administration (FDA) approved a new drug, rasagiline, for the treatment of Parkinson's disease (PD). Rasagiline, which will be sold under the name of Azilect° in the United States, is taken once a day. The manufacturer, Teva Pharmaceuticals, intends to have two strengths of this drug available for sale in the US later this year.

The FDA approved rasagiline as a stand-alone treatment for early PD and in combination with levodopa, a commonly used drug to treat PD, for the signs and symptoms of moderate to advanced PD. These approvals were based on the results of three clinical studies.

The first study included 404 participants who had early PD and were not taking any dopamine-like drugs for the treatment of PD. The study lasted for 26 weeks. The results showed that rasagiline was better than placebo at controlling the symptoms of PD, as measured by the Unified Parkinson Disease Rating Scale (UPDRS). The UPDRS is a tool that doctors often use in research studies to measure the effects of PD.

A total of 1,159 people with moderate to severe PD participated in the second two studies. These people were taking levodopa and had motor fluctuations, dyskinesias, or both. They kept a diary at home and recorded the amount of

---

[12] nwpf@nwpf.org or http://nwpf.nwpf.org

"off" time that they had each day. Both studies found that the addition of rasagiline to the subjects' usual medications **reduced the amount of off time**, as compared with before they started taking rasagiline. In addition, some people were able to **decrease their dose of levodopa**.

Additional studies will be conducted to evaluate the impact of dietary tyramine on people taking rasagiline (see the information below on monoamine oxidase (MAO-B) inhibitors) and whether taking rasagiline increases a person's risk of developing melanoma. In the studies of rasagiline that have been completed, the rate of melanoma was slightly higher in those taking rasagiline, but it is not clear whether this was due to the drug or happened by chance and was not related to the drug. For now, people taking rasagiline should follow a diet that **does not include foods that contain tyramine** and should undergo regularly scheduled examinations of their skin to look for melanomas.

Monoamine Oxidase Inhibitors

Azilect is in a class of drugs known as *monoamine oxidase inhibitors* (MAOIs). These drugs affect chemicals in the brain known as *monoamines*--serotonin, dopamine, and norepinephrine. Monoamines are involved in the transmission of messages between nerve cells. Dopamine is particularly important in regulating messages related to movement. People with PD have a decreased amount of dopamine in their brains.

After monoamines perform their jobs as messengers, they are broken down by a type of protein known as an *oxidase*. Rasagiline, like other MAOIs, limits, or is an *inhibitor* of oxidation, (which is the process of combining oxygen with some other substance). Because they inhibit oxidation, MAOIs **increase the level of monoamines, including dopamine, in the brain.**

Unfortunately, MAOIs also inhibit or prevent the breakdown of a naturally occurring substance known as tyramine. When tyramine builds up in the body, it can cause **extremely high blood pressure,** leading to rupture of blood vessels in the brain or even death. Many prescription and over-the-counter medications, such as antidepressants and cough-and-cold medicines, and dietary supplements contain tyramine or also interfere with the breakdown of tyramine. Therefore, if you are taking rasagiline, make sure that you are aware of these substances and that every healthcare provider who cares for you, including the person administering your anesthesia, if you are having an operation, knows that you are taking an MAOI.

A wide variety of foods also contain tyramine, and the level of tyramine increases in protein-based or processed foods as the protein breaks down. Eating the freshest possible meats and other protein-based foods is very important. Therefore, it's a good idea if you are taking an MAOI, to **eat only food that is freshly prepared**--let someone else finish off the leftovers, and you may want to steer clear of the buffet line at a restaurant. Some foods should be limited because they contain small amounts of tyramine, and others should be avoided completely. Be sure to check with your doctor for a complete listing of foods and medications that you should avoid. People with liver problems should also not take MAOIs. (Google Tyramine, for more information)

People who take MAOIs should be aware of the symptoms of high levels of tyramine, including severe headache, blurred vision, difficulty thinking, seizures, chest pain, unexplained nausea or vomiting, or signs or symptoms of a stroke. Patients and caregivers should seek immediate medical attention for patients who develop any severe headache or other atypical or unusual symptoms not previously experienced

Alternative and Adjunctive Therapies

Extract from SPRING Times No. 32, July 2004 Page 12[13]:
By Michael Kelly
The following is a continuation in the Matrix series, the first of which appeared in ST 30, under the title: A research matrix for PD. It details possible approaches in treating PD, this block within the matrix being classified as (relatively) low cost and having a moderate time frame for making useful progress. Due to space limitations the article is necessarily restricted to a brief mention of various therapies. Further information is available from the author.

Conventional pharmacological treatment of Pd, often extending over decades, involves potent drugs acting on the central nervous system. Together with considerable benefits,

[13] www.spring.parkinsons.org.uk
SPRING: 99 Park Lane, Sandbach CW11 IEJ, England.
Phone 01403 823 947

this entails serious, well-documented side effects. Moreover, though many problems associated with Pd are not drug responsive, non-pharmacological treatments are often mentioned, almost as an afterthought, in many publications dealing with treatment of Pd. Increases in dose and addition of other drugs, to counteract diminishing response or to treat side effects, seldom provide more than a transient benefit, followed by more complications, creating a vicious circle.

By placing too much emphasis on drug therapy, patients are likely to become unduly dependent, both on their medication and on others, adopting a passive role and not retaining the responsibility for keeping fit and maintaining a sense of well-being, by their own efforts.

Alternative and adjunctive therapies that can help to maintain an element of control, **postponing or reducing the use of drugs**, while holding the therapeutic window open for as long as possible.

In a simplified picture, such therapies can be divided into two categories, namely:
1. those whose effectiveness is largely or wholly beyond doubt
2. those whose effectiveness is open to doubt or remains controversial

Examples in the first category include

- *Movement exercises and gymnastics of various kinds*
- *Zeptor/CHI Massage*
- *Swimming*
- *Speech therapy*
- *Ergo therapy*
- *Relaxation exercises*

Exercise, in all its various forms, is undoubtedly one of the most important elements in adjunctive therapy for Pd. Apart from improving general health; it creates **a sense of well-being, reduces complications of immobility, helps to maintain functional facilities, promotes coordination and balance and improves sleep,** to name but some benefits. Swimming, speech therapy, physiotherapy and the like all have an assured role in helping to counteract the effects of Pd."

The following comments will be confined to a brief description of a recent development referred to as **Zeptor.**

Charcot, in 1904, observed that Pd symptoms were alleviated by train journeys. Rail travel involved considerably more jolting and jerking than it does now. This observation by the eminent French neurologist finds expression in a new development, by the Sports Medicine department at Frankfurt University. Zeptor is a device designed to stimulate motor responses, by using multi-dimensional mechanical oscillations programmed, in a random sequence. Two foot plates on which the patient stands, execute complex motions, at adjustable amplitudes and frequencies. The device as it was designed originally was used to mimic the sensations of downhill skiing, for top-class alpine skiers, creating perturbations simulating skiing over rough terrain.

In treating Pd patients, a frequency of 6 Hz is usually used for a 1-2 minute period, repeated 5 times, with amplitude selected to suit the individual. The range extends from gentle vibrations to extremely pronounced shaking.

Tests done with over 1000 patients in Germany and Spain point to an improvement in symptoms in about 80% of cases, lasting from 2 hours up to 48 hours. The device is relatively expensive, and is more suited to neurologists' practices or meeting centre installation than to home use. It is safe and well tolerated by the vast majority of patients. A small number have complained of nausea or seasickness like symptoms.

While Zeptor does not represent exercise in the classical sense, it does appear to offer exercise-like benefits and is establishing itself in a niche role in Pd therapy in Germany.

Examples in the second category include:

- *Acupuncture*
- *Transcranial magnetic stimulation (rTMS)*
- *Aromatherapy*
- *Homeopathy*
- *Reiki/Tuina/Johrei*

Patients are often encouraged to believe that one or other therapy will solve their problems and are willing to part with considerable sums of money in a search, which is often ultimately disappointing. This is not to say that some may experience benefits from alternative therapies, be they placebo-related or the result of other factors. The following comments are confined to acupuncture and rTMS.

The effectiveness of acupuncture remains controversial as a treatment for Pd, despite its widespread use in Western countries for a whole range of conditions. The literature contains very considerable numbers of reports of studies and trials specifically as it relates to Pd. Acupuncture, of course, does not lend itself to blinded studies. Yet perusal of the literature leaves one more confused than before and does little to remove doubts about the efficacy of this therapy on a wider basis.

In a recent paper, by Schuman L.M. and co-workers[14] a broad battery of tests was used to assess the effectiveness of acupuncture, including Sickness Impact Profile (SIP), UPDRS, Hoehn and Yahr (H&Y), Schwab and England (S&E), Beck Anxiety Inventory (BAI), Beck Depression Inventory (BDI) and qualitative motor tests and a patient questionnaire designed for the study. Following a significant number of treatment sessions, no significant difference was found in any of the scores except one. The only variable showing any improvement was the sleep and rest category of SIP. However, 85% of patients reported subjective improvement of individual symptoms including tremor, walking, handwriting, slowness, pain, sleep, depression and anxiety in the patient questionnaire, something not reflected in the objective scientific Assessment criteria. While this outcome may not correlate with the results obtained in all studies, it is rather typical of findings in many. As there are essentially no doubts about safety and tolerability of acupuncture when carried out by a competent acupuncturist, the method is suitable for trial to determine if it helps with symptoms in individual cases.

Transcranial Magnetic Stimulation (TMS) in its current form has been in use for nearly 20 years[15]. The technique involves induction of electrical fields in the brain by passing a current through a coil or coils placed over the head, using rapidly changing, very short duration pulses. A train of such pulses applied to a particular brain area at a specific frequency is referred to as repetitive TMS (rTMS). A range of stimulation frequencies (most studies used 5-8 Hz), impulse durations and field intensities (from pica Tesla levels up to 5 Teslas) give rise to an array of different stimulation effects.

---

[14] *Schuman L.M., et al, "Acupuncture therapy for the symptoms of Parkinson's disease", Movement Disorders, July 2002; 17 (4); p 799-802.*
[15] *Baker AT, Jalinous R, Freeston IL, Non-Invasive magnetic stimulation of human motor cortex, Lancet 1985; 1; p 1106-07*

rTms has been shown to be capable of modulating cortical activity, whereby pathological over- or under-activity can be "normalized"[16]. Whether this takes place via long-term potentiation or depression of synapses is unclear. rTMS has been used extensively in the treatment of depression and some tantalizing results have been obtained in the treatment of Pd:

Pascual-Leone and co-workers have published data with positive results as have Strafella and co-workers[17] and Mally and Stone[18]. Sandyk, working in the US, has been using rTMS for over 10 years, in treating Pd and has published extensively on the subject, claiming much success[19]. Henneberg and co-workers have tested over 200 patients, in the Bad Nauheim Parkinson clinic, achieving an average improvement of 32% in UPDRS III. In some individual cases, the improvement has been very marked and has persisted over several months. However, other studies have not shown any beneficial effects., so that the evidence for a clear therapeutic effect is clouded and it seems premature to give rTMS a therapeutic role without further testing. There appears to be a marked variability in outcome across patients, this coupled with the range of variables used in testing at different locations makes it difficult to reach a firm conclusion about the therapy.

The technique is non-invasive and painless and found to be generally safe, when measures are taken to exclude patients, who may be susceptible to epileptic seizures.

Depression: An international survey on factors impacting quality of life in Pd, brings out the point very clearly that depression plays a major role in Pd. The report of the Global Pd survey, extending to 1020 patients in six countries published in December 2001, stated "...Currently, successful management of Pd is predominantly measured by the control

[16] *Kobayashi M., Pascual-Leone A,.; Transcranial magnetic stimulation in neurology; Vol 2, 3; 2003; p 145-156.*
[17] *Strafella AP et al, Repetitive transcranial magnetic stimulation of the human prefrontal cortex induces dopamine release in the caudate nucleus Journal Neuroscience, 2001; 21; RC 157*
[18] *Mally J., Stone T.W., Improvement in Parkinsonian symptoms after repetitive transcranial magnetic stimulation, J Neurtol. Science; 162; 1999; p 179-184.*
[19] *Sandyk R., Parkinsonism microglia reversal by treatment with weak electromagnetic fields, Intl. Jour. Neuroscience, 1995; 81; p 873-93.*

of motor symptoms and management protocols, therefore, focus on drug therapy"[20]. High levels of depression were found in Pd and this was found to have a significant effect on HRQL. Rather surprisingly, patients rarely report depression, although the Beck Depression Inventory (BDI) assesses more than 50% as depressed.

The report goes on to demonstrate that factors, other than disease severity and medication, contribute significantly to health-related quality of life (HRQL) in Pd. This finding, supported by other studies from Finland and the UK, indicates that depression needs to be put very high in the list of priorities in clinical management of Pd. This calls for a different, more innovative and more holistic approach to testing Pd, than is oftentimes currently the case. Psychosocial adjustment, emotional well-being and maintenance of functional capabilities, all need to be nurtured, in order for patients to remain optimistic and develop better coping strategies.

Conclusions

Being healthy is not a scientifically or legally defined condition; it is an emotionally perceived state. In as far as this state can be influenced or modified by the individual concerned, the possibility exists of being able to exercise a degree of control on how the disease affects quality of life.

It is not uncommon for mildly affected patients to suffer severe psychological anxiety while others with pronounced disabilities live quite happy, well-adjusted lives.

Alternative and adjunctive therapies can play a major role in creating a favorable environment to foster an attractive quality of life. A shift of emphasis **away from drugs, towards adjunctive therapies** would enhance a sense of well-being, giving patients an incentive to adopt a more active role in managing their disease.

---

[20] *Factors impacting on Quality of Life in Parkinson's Disease; Results from an International Survey, Movement Disorders; 17; 1, 2002, p60-67.*

The following supportive information on alternative and adjunctive therapies was supplied by the *Parkinson's Post, Published by the Northwest Parkinson's Foundation.*

Where Martial Arts Meets Meditation, Invigoration Follows
David Ball

Herald Tribune.com - Sarasota resident Menachem Hirmes walked slowly, hunched over and shaking -- some of the more visible symptoms of Parkinson's disease.

But for 45 serene minutes, his body calmed as he and 20 other tai chi enthusiasts moved and breathed in unison. They performed a Kung Fu-like ballet using moves named "white stork spreads wings," "go back to ward off monkey," and "carry tiger to mountain."

Four years ago, Hirmes watched as his wife used tai chi to alleviate the pain in her rotator cuff and hip joints. Now he hopes this combination of martial arts and meditation can improve his quality of life.

"So far, I love it. It's helped my body to relax," said Hirmes, who has practiced for two years. "I'm hoping it will help my posture and balance."

The largely unstudied health benefits of tai chi are the main reason why nearly 150 full-time and seasonal residents have joined the Sarasota chapter of the Taoist Tai Chi Society.

The chapter is one of the largest in Florida and an important fundraising and outreach center within the International Taoist Tai Chi Society, which includes 40,000 members in 30 U.S. states and 26 countries from Europe to Asia to Latin America.

Surveys show that as many as 3 million people practice tai chi in the United States.

This year, the international society purchased a 5,000-sq-ft former church, on South Lockwood Ridge Road, to be the Sarasota chapter's new home. The center opened May 15, becoming only the sixth permanent Taoist Tai Chi center in the U.S.

"We've moved from rental to rental, but this gives us a permanent place and room to grow," Sarasota chapter founder Mickey Hopkins said. "In Sarasota in particular, there's a great deal of curiosity and awareness of alternative medicine and different philosophical teachings."

Taoist Tai Chi began in 1970 in Montreal, Canada. A Chinese Taoist monk named Moy Lin-shin began teaching a form of internal (non-combative) martial arts combined with Taoist teachings of compassion, moderation, humility and a spiritual connection to nature and the universe.

What began as classes in outdoor parking lots grew in popularity and spread as students relocated.

The movement reached Florida in the early 1980s, and the Taoist Tai Chi Society of Florida was incorporated in 1985.

The Sarasota chapter began in the early 1990s, when Hopkins began taking tai chi classes in St. Petersburg. Within three years, Hopkins was certified as an instructor.

Like all chapters, the Taoist Tai Chi Society of Sarasota is a nonprofit run by an elected council and supported by donations.

"It's completely volunteer supported. The only paid persons are our executive directors in Tallahassee and in Canada", Sarasota chapter president Debbie Gates said.

Lin-shin claimed his early studies in China cured his various sicknesses, and he focused his later teachings on the health benefits of Taoist Tai Chi.

He developed a set of 108 specific moves, that emphasize balance, flexibility, meditation and stimulation of internal organs. Those moves are the only moves performed by Taoist Tai Chi groups.

While the health benefits of tai chi are widely described by practitioners and instructors, there are few long-term and comprehensive medical studies to back up these claims.

The National Center, for Complementary and Alternative Medicine, has collected studies on the effect of tai chi on cardiovascular disease, fall prevention, osteoporosis, arthritis, chronic heart failure, cancer survivors, depression in the elderly and fibromyalgia.

One study on the immune response to varicella-zoster virus (which causes shingles) in 2007 stated that tai chi might strengthen the immune system in older adults. In 2008, a review of published research found that tai chi reduced participants' blood pressure in 22 of 26 studies.

However, "in general, studies of tai chi have been small, or they have had design limitations that may limit their conclusions," the center's website states. "The cumulative evidence suggests that additional research is warranted and needed before tai chi can be widely recommended as an effective therapy."

But recently, Harvard University researcher Catherine Kerr has contended that tai chi benefits are real -- especially for older people, too frail for robust aerobic conditioning and for those suffering from impaired balance, joint stiffness, or poor kinesthetic awareness.

The Sarasota chapter offers a "health recovery" class in which participants perform moves, while seated in wheelchairs. "We had a lady walking for the first time in 12 years," Hopkins said.

The Hope of Music's Healing Powers
Melissa Healy

The Los Angeles Times - Yes, yes, it hath charms to soothe a savage breast (or beast, if you prefer to repeat a common mistake). But researchers are finding that music may be an effective balm for many other afflictions: the isolation of conditions such as autism and Alzheimer's disease, the disability that results from stroke, the physical stress of entering the world too early.

The hope of music's curative powers has spawned a community in the United States of some 5,000 registered music therapists, who have done post-college study in psychology and music to gain certification. Active primarily in hospitals, nursing homes, special needs classrooms and rehabilitation units, music therapists aim to soothe, stimulate and support the development or recovery of abilities lost to illness or injury.

While music therapists use a mix of improvisation and proven techniques to help patients, neuroscientists are looking to uncover the scientific basis for music's healing powers. They are trying to understand how music can help rewire a brain affected by illness or injury, or provide a work-around for injured or underperforming brain regions.

By doing so, they hope to better identify which patients might respond best to music and what musical techniques might best help them to regain lost or compromised function.

"Music might provide an alternative entry point to the brain, because it can unlock so many different doors into an injured or ill brain", said Dr. Gottfried Schlaug, a Harvard University neurologist. Pitch, harmony, melody, rhythm and emotion - all components of music - engage different regions of the brain.

"And many of those same regions are also important in speech, movement and social interaction. If a disease or trauma has disabled a brain region needed for such functions, music can sometimes get in through a back door and coax them out by another route", Schlaug says: "In a sense, we're using musical tools to particularly engage certain parts of the brain and then teach the brain new tricks - new tools - to overcome an impairment," he says.

Neuroscientists are exploring the role of music in treatment of some of the following:

Speech: For about 1 in 5 patients who suffer a stroke, difficulty with speech - aphasia - is a lingering effect. Schlaug and other researchers have found that by practicing to express themselves with a simple form of singing - something that sounds almost like Gregorian chant - aphasic stroke victims significantly improved the fluency of their speech, compared with patients, whose speech therapy did not include singing.

Schlaug says, "it appears that the 'melodic intonation therapy', as it's termed, bypassed the stroke damage done to speech centers in aphasic patients' left brain hemisphere. Instead, it engaged and recruited areas of their healthy right hemispheres that were capable of - though not generally used for - word acquisition and speech".

The patients tapped along as they sang, which also seemed to engage a broad network in the brain, involved in detecting and reproducing rhythm. Such strategies, it turned out, allowed aphasics' words to come out.

Movement: If you're old enough, recall John Travolta walking down the street to the song "Stayin' Alive" in the opening scene of "Saturday Night Fever." Now imagine a patient with Parkinson's disease, a degenerative brain condition that affects the initiation and smooth completion of movement. Here's where music's rhythmic qualities appear to get in the back door of a patient's brain and provide a work-around to brain functions degraded by Parkinson's. By engaging the network of regions that perceive and anticipate rhythm, music with a steady, predictable beat, can be used to cue the brain's motor regions to initiate walking.

Once off the dime, a Parkinson's patient can use the music's beat to maintain a steady, rhythmic gait, like John Travolta.

"It works well and it works instantaneously, and it's hard to think of any medication that has this effect," Schlaug says.

Neuroscientists suspect that music may work in much the same way for stutterers, who can experience difficulties initiating speech and maintaining a steady flow of words. Case studies have long observed that when stutterers sing, their halting speech patterns disappear. Music's predictable beats may help them initiate speech and continue fluently.

Reading: Research suggests that people with dyslexia, or difficulty reading, also fare poorly on tests of auditory processing. Their timing is also poor. They have difficulty filtering out unwanted background noise and "tuning in" to sounds — such as a teacher's instruction — that they want to hear. Intensive music instruction has been found to improve those skills, and with them, some skills related to reading.

Memory: The progressive degeneration of memory in Alzheimer's disease cannot be reversed or slowed by any intervention. But music can temporarily unlock memories for patients, who have lost their grip on nearly every other detail of their daily life and relationships.

Patients in the depths of Alzheimer's and other dementias regularly respond to — and even play and sing — music from their distant past, without missing a word or a note. Nursing homes have seized upon that fact, exposing residents to the songs of their childhoods or courtship years to help reunite spouses, in dancing and singing, and try to coax dementia sufferers from their isolation. One study even found that dementia patients allowed to punch a button on a robot and hear a familiar song experienced improved mood, function and performance on musical memory games.

Preemies' weight gain: An Israeli study, published December in the journal Pediatrics, found that playing Mozart quietly, in neonatal intensive care units, supported the weight gain of premature infants, by slowing their rate of energy expenditure. Babies exposed over two days to 30 minutes of music (drawn from, yes, an Israeli "Mozart for Baby" CD) slowed their metabolisms, helping to accelerate their growth.

Whether Mozart is worth using routinely in neonatal care units, the researchers say, will take further study.

Researchers Unlocking Learning
Strategies in Parkinson's Patients

PhysOrg.com - The research, published recently in the Journal of Neurophysiology shows that patients are better able to learn tasks, necessary for adapting to their disease—how to button their shirt differently or how to use a cane or walker for steadiness, for example—when they are not medicated, during early stages of the learning process. This is particularly true for early-stage Parkinson's patients.

Most Parkinson's patients suffer from four main symptoms: Tremors, stiffness or rigidity of the limbs and trunk, slow movement, and impaired balance and coordination. As these symptoms become more pronounced and the disease progresses, patients may have difficulty walking, talking, or completing other simple tasks and often require physical therapy to help them learn how to manage.

Previous research showed that Parkinson's patients performed learning tasks better, off medications, than on medications, but U-M researcher Rachael Seidler was particularly interested in the effects of medication, early in the learning process. Parkinson's disease often affects the upper region of the brain first, gradually working its way down to the lower region of the brain, where learning sequences of actions takes place. Normally, the brain relies on the chemical dopamine, for communication between its parts. In people with Parkinson's disease, reduced levels of dopamine hamper such communication. Several drugs currently used in Parkinson's treatment boost dopamine, but some of these medications can "overdose" unaffected regions of the brain, interfering with learning.

Seidler and colleagues, hypothesized that patients would learn new sequences better and faster when "off" medication, early in the learning process. The researchers expected this to be particularly true of patients, with early-stage Parkinson's, because the lower parts of their brains would net yet be affected by the disease.

The study tested Parkinson's patients over two days, both on and off medication. Healthy people with no neurological impairments were also tested for comparison. The Parkinson's patients stopped taking their regular dose of dopamine-boosting medication 12 to18 hours before testing.

All subjects in the study were given a learning task that involved pressing a key, in response to something flashed on a computer screen. Participants also were instructed to press the appropriate button as fast as possible, when an "X" appeared, and to press the key in a specific sequential pattern. Different sequences were tested over the two-day period, to assess new sequence-learning behaviors, the idea being that as patients learned the sequences, they would become faster at pressing the appropriate buttons.

Seidler and colleagues, found that Parkinson's patients, off medication, responded exactly like healthy controls, while patients, on medication, showed clear signs of impairment. The researchers concluded that **dopamine overdosing in healthy parts of the brain indeed hampers early stages of sequence learning.**

"Normally you would think, giving people a drug to replace dopamine, would improve motor skills—and it does to an extent," said Seidler, a professor at the School of Kinesiology and Department of Psychology and lead author of the study. "But there are other behaviors, where the brain relies on dopamine as a neurotransmitter, that is not affected in the early stages of the disease. Dopamine replacement medications are not spatially selective—they go everywhere in the brain. If you have too much dopamine going into healthy parts of the brain, it can cause behavioral impairments, as we witnessed in our study."

Seidler and colleagues hope the results of this study will lead to new treatment strategies for Parkinson's patients, specifically more targeted drug delivery.

Index